HOSPITALS

What They Are and How They Work

Second Edition

I. Donald Snook, Jr.

President
Presbyterian Medical Center of Philadelphia
Philadelphia, Pennsylvania

AN ASPEN PUBLICATION®
Aspen Publishers, Inc.
Gaithersburg, Maryland
1992

Library of Congress Cataloging-in-Publication Data

Snook, I. Donald
Hospitals: what they are and how they work /
I. Donald Snook, Jr.—2nd ed.
p. cm.
Includes bibliographical references and index.
ISBN: 0-8342-0247-6
1. Hospitals. 2. Hospitals—Administration.
3. Hospitals—United States. I. Title.
[DNLM: 1. Hospital Administration—United States.
2. Hospitals—United States. WX 100 S673h]
RA963.S57 1991
362.1'1'068—dc20
DNLM/DLC
for Library of Congress
91-18269
CIP

Editorial Services: Becky Mangus
Lisa Hajjar

Library of Congress Catalog Card Number: 91-18269
ISBN: 0-8342-0247-6

Printed in the United States of America

1 2 3 4 5

Table of Contents

Introduction

Hospitals are among the most complex institutions in our society. They are an integral part of America. Hospitals touch all of our lives. Over the years their basic mission has evolved to the point where they are today the focal point of a community's medical care.

The principal objective of this book is to offer the reader an understanding of the organization, internal operations, and functions of the hospital. In examining the hospital, the book takes a general overview approach. The community general hospital was the model used in most of the book's illustrations and examples. One of the purposes of the work is to acquaint the reader with the methods and systems most often used within the medium-sized community general hospital. Specifically, the book addresses these questions: How does a hospital function? What are the major components that make up a hospital? Who are the personnel and staff that run the hospital? What are their roles in the organization? Who has the power within the hospital? How does a hospital grow? Where does the hospital fit into the larger medical care system?

The book is divided into several parts that follow a logical sequence. It starts with the hospital's early beginning. It then goes inside the hospital, starting with management, followed by a description of the services offered and the departments that provide those services. Next is a discussion of how a hospital evaluates its care. The book concludes with some thoughts on how hospitals grow and a description of the elements of a health care system.

Part I

Where Did the Hospital Come from?

Chapter 1

A Brief History

Key Terms

Hospitium • Council of Nicaea • Almshouse • Pennsylvania Hospital • Dispensary • Transplantations • Spare parts medicine • Hill-Burton legislation • Medicare and Medicaid legislation • Diagnostic Related Groups

THE BEGINNING (BIRTH OF CHRIST–MIDDLE AGES)

It is difficult in the twentieth century to imagine that the modern skyscraper medical centers that serve the health care needs of our sprawling communities really started as something quite different. The word *hospital* comes from the Greek word *hospitium*, a word that is mentioned frequently in the literature from the fifth century A.D. onward. In early history, hospitium meant something quite different from our modern hospital term. Hospitium was a place for the reception of strangers and pilgrims.

Following the birth of Christianity, Christians were encouraged to make pilgrimages to the many holy places of the Middle East. For several centuries, travelers from Western Europe made their way into this part of the world. Many of these pilgrims traveled without money, believing that they would receive assistance on their way from other accommodating Christians. Many hospitals (in the Greek sense of hospitium) were established, particularly in remote and dangerous places. For example, to house the pilgrimaging Christians, it was common for well-to-do Christians to bequeath resources in order to provide the travelers with necessary services. These services were extended as tangible gifts in the spirit of Christ. Hospitals were also established by the Christian church as instruments for the propagation of the faith—as living testimonies to the healing mission of Jesus.

3

Many of the great hospitals can be traced to the period directly following the Council of Nicaea in 325 A.D., when the bishops of the church were instructed to go out into every cathedral city in Christendom and start a hospital. The momentum for the founding of hospitiums on the way to the holy city was assumed and aided by several knightly orders that took on the responsibility of establishing and maintaining these wayside places of rest. The best known of these knightly orders was the Knights of St. John, or the Hospitalers.

The oldest operative hospital in the Western world today is the Hotel Dieu in Paris.[1] This hospital was established around 600 A.D. by Saint Landry, the Bishop of Paris. Even by current standards, this early French hospital could truly be called a medical center, since it has always embraced many of the varied activities necessary to care for the sick.

Though the Crusades gave impetus to the development of hospitals along the road to the holy land, the travelers brought back to England and other parts of Western Europe the disease of leprosy, which until the time of the Crusades had not been experienced in epidemic proportions in either England or Central Europe. About 1100 A.D., to cope with the spreading leprosy invasion, some 200 hospitals, called "lazar houses," were established in England specifically for the care of lepers. This is a large number of hospitals considering that the entire English population at this time was only about three million.[2]

EARLY AMERICAN HOSPITALS (FOUNDING OF THE NEW WORLD–WORLD WAR II)

With the exploration of the New World on the North American continent, various French, Spanish, and English colonies were founded. However, none of these settlements brought about a lasting system of hospitals. Institutions for the sick at that time were simply temporary makeshift arrangements set up to care for specific illnesses.

Cortez is credited with establishing the first permanent, solid hospital structure on the North American continent in 1524. The Jesus of Nazareth Hospital is still functioning in Mexico City; it stands as a magnificent example of Spanish architectural genius and a monument to Cortez and the Spanish conquerors of Mexico.

The first American hospitals can be traced to the early eighteenth century. These were hastily structured arrangements, built primarily to confine contagious diseases during epidemics. They were founded mainly in seaport towns, such as New York, Philadelphia, Charleston, and Newport. It was not until the eighteenth century that attempts were made to provide continuous service in the form of hospitals. These institutions were called almshouses. They were established primarily for the urban poor and were a direct result of urban crowding. The first American almshouse was founded in 1713 by William Penn in Philadelphia. It was originally restricted to indigent Quakers, but in 1782, a new building, constructed to serve all the urban poor, opened in Philadelphia.

Pennsylvania Hospital in Philadelphia, established in 1751, is considered to be the oldest voluntary hospital in the country. Its mission—to serve the sick poor— began to emerge as a result of the efforts of Benjamin Franklin and Dr. Thomas Bond. They championed the cause of Pennsylvania Hospital since little medical attention was provided for the city's poor and mentally ill, while well-to-do residents received medical care in their homes. Pennsylvania Hospital and the hospitals that followed were established in the same general pattern used for such hospitals in England. Pennsylvania Hospital was built with funds appropriated by the provincial legislature and matched by public subscriptions. As patients recuperated, they were required to help pay for lengthy stays by serving food to other patients or scrubbing floors.

It is important to remember that these early hospitals were devoted generally to the care of the sick, but they were primarily used by the homeless and the poor sick. Many physicians did not make use of these hospitals for their private patients. In fact, as late as 1908, the Massachusetts General Hospital in Boston still cared only for the poor, and physicians were not permitted to charge fees to their patients.

These hospitals also faced an influx of mentally ill patients. The first mental hospital in the United States was constructed in 1772 in Williamsburg, Virginia and carried the descriptive name of Eastern Lunatic Asylum.[3] The humanistic treatment of mental illness within a medical framework was introduced in France by Philipee Pinel in 1796. Pinel's effort was paralleled by Dr. Benjamin Rush in the United States during the same time period.

The first Catholic hospital in the United States was founded in 1828 by the Daughters of Charity of St. Vincent DePaul in St. Louis.[4] It was called the DePaul Hospital. Eight years later, the St. Joseph Infirmary opened in Louisville, Kentucky as a shelter for orphans and plague victims; it was staffed by the Sisterhood Charity of Nazareth. The reputation of these early American hospitals was not enviable. Because the death rate in these hospitals was staggeringly high, due in part to severe epidemics, people considered them a last resort.

Rapidly growing urban centers gave great impetus to the expansion of the American hospital. The need for teaching and research facilities led to the establishment of the urban teaching centers and medical school hospitals that continue to be important today in the training of medical students and physicians.

One of the major turning points in the history of hospitals came with the discovery of ether as an anesthetic. The discovery of ether is usually attributed to W.T.G. Morton, a Georgia dentist, who arranged for the first hospital surgical procedure using ether in 1846. Crawford Long later reported that he had used ether during an operation in 1842; however, he did not publish reports of his work until after Morton's discovery was already known. The use of ether somewhat reduced the public's fear of hospitals and also accounted for a dramatic increase in surgery.

In the latter part of the nineteenth century, following the work of Pasteur in bacteriology and Lister in antiseptic surgery, the hospital began to emerge as a place to get well. With the introduction of sulfa drugs in the 1930s and penicillin in the 1940s, it became possible to do surgery with considerably less infection mortality. From that point on, the hospital began to acquire a better image as a place for citizens to go to receive treatment and to recover.

Just as the poor sick spurred the founding of hospitals, the poor also stimulated the origin of organized ambulatory or outpatient care. A Protestant French doctor, Théophraste Renaudot, established a free consultation service outside the hospital for the sick poor in Paris in 1630.[5] In 1641, the dispensary of drugs was added. "Dispensaries," as they were called, also spread to the New World to serve the urban poor. By the end of the 19th century, there was a decline in the number of dispensaries as hospitals began to develop organized outpatient departments or what we have grown to know as hospital clinics.

THE MODERN ERA (POST WORLD WAR II–PRESENT)

With the public health movement of the 19th century and the expansion of medical technology following World War II, health threats changed. The previous acute disease epidemics were replaced by chronic and debilitative diseases. The growing and formidable technology helped to combat some of these illnesses. For example, in 1954, the first successful kidney transplantation took place and with that the modern era of "spare parts medicine" began. As an illustration of the continuing technical revolution in human organ transplantation, we witnessed the first heart transplant and the first liver transplant in 1967; the first heart-lung transplant in 1981 and the first permanent artificial heart transplant in 1982. Today, we continue to experience an increase in "spare parts medicine." In 1989, 8,886 kidneys, 2,160 livers, 1,673 hearts, 417 pancreases, 89 lungs, and 70 heart-lungs were transplanted.

In the mainstream of medicine's advancing technology, our nation's hospitals are also affected by intense government involvement and regulation. Ever since the Commonwealth of Pennsylvania gave the Pennsylvania Hospital a grant in the 1750s, government has provided assistance to our hospitals. In 1948, the Hospital Survey and Construction Act, known as the Hill-Burton legislation was passed. This legislation provided hospitals—which accepted a commitment to care for the poor—with funds for construction. In 1960, Congress passed the Kerr-Mills Bill which provided joint federal and state assistance for the medically indigent. But the most formidable government involvement occurred in 1965, when the Social Security Amendments, Public Laws 89–97, were passed creating Medicare and

Medicaid. In 1972, Congress passed additional Social Security Amendments which allowed for the funding of dialysis and transplants for individuals with end-stage renal disease. In 1983, Congress passed legislation targeted to control the ever-increasing costs of the Medicare program by establishing Medicare's Diagnostic Related Groups (DRGs), a prospective payment system (PPS). These are just some of the examples of government's increasing involvement in hospital affairs. Only the future will show whether hospitals' preoccupation with governmental regulation, which some equate with bureaucratic red tape, will affect the cost or quality of patient care.

As we have seen, early American hospitals drew much of their heritage from European hospitals. But the modern American hospital developed rapidly and quite differently from its early counterparts.

Hospitals began to care for the sick almost incidentally. The earliest hospitals were interested in pilgrims, the indigent, and plague victims. Later they became institutions where people from all parts of society could come for diagnosis and recovery.

The hospital as an institution has been dynamic; it exists today because it meets the needs of the people it serves. Today's hospitals continue to write history by reacting to the changing needs of society for better technologies, new services and greater access.

NOTES

1. Charles V. Letourneau, "History of Hospitals, Part I," *Hospital Management,* March 1959, p. 58.

2. Charles V. Letourneau, "History of Hospitals, Part II," *Hospital Management,* April 1959, p. 52.

3. Malcolm MacEachern, *Hospital Organization and Management* (Chicago, Ill.: Physicians' Record Co., 1957), p. 16.

4. Robin O'Connor, "American Hospitals: The First 200 Years," *Hospitals, JAHA,* p. 67.

5. Milton I. Roemer, "Ambulatory Health Services in America: Past, Present and Future," (Rockville, MD: Aspen Publishers, Inc., 1981), p. 15.

6. "Business Facts," *AHA News,* 9 July 1990, p. 7.

Chapter 2

Today's Hospital

Key Terms

Classification of hospitals • Community hospitals • Hospital beds • Outpatient care • Hospital expenditures • Hospital revenues

HOW BIG IS THE HOSPITAL INDUSTRY?

There are 6,780 hospitals in the United States with a total capacity of 1.25 million hospital beds.[1] As a measure of the hospital industry's output, these institutions handled some 34.1 million admissions and more than 336 million outpatient visits in 1988 alone.[2] The hospital industry represents a mix of public and private sectors. Hospitals can be classified in several ways, and they may be categorized as community or noncommunity. Community hospitals represent the majority of American hospitals. Noncommunity hospitals include federal hospitals as well as certain specialty hospitals.

There are 5,533 community hospitals in this country (Table 2.1),[3] approximately half of which are in rural areas. Community hospitals may be classified in several ways. One key index used to measure or classify a hospital is the institution's number of inpatient beds, often referred to as the hospital's bed size. Community hospitals may also be classified as investor-owned (proprietary) or not-for-profit (voluntary) institutions. Although the number of investor-owned hospitals continues to increase, in 1987 they comprised only a small minority of community hospitals. Hospitals may also be organized as either general hospitals or specialty hospitals. General hospitals see a wide variety of medical problems. Specialty hospitals (e.g., a children's hospital or a psychiatric hospital) limit their care to specific illnesses or patients.

Table 2-1 Selected Measures in Community Hospitals, 1979 and 1988–89

Measure	Year			Percent Change*	
	1979	1988	1989	1979–89	1988–89
Hospitals	5,842	5,533	5,455	− 6.6%	−1.4%
Beds (in thousands)	984	947	933	− 5.1%	−1.4%
Average number of beds per hospital	168	171	171	1.6%	0.0%
Admissions (in thousands)	35,099	31,453	31,116	−11.3%	−1.1%
Average daily census (in thousands)	727	620	618	−15.1%	−0.4%
Average length of stay (in days)	7.6	7.2	7.2	− 4.1%	0.4%
Inpatient days (in thousands)	265,207	226,875	225,437	−15.0%	−0.6%
Occupancy percent	73.9	65.5	66.2	−10.5%	1.0%
Surgical operations (in thousands)	18,269	21,411	21,340	16.8%	−0.3%
Bassinets (in thousands)	77	70	69	−10.2%	−1.3%
Births (in thousands)	3,287	3,706	3,831	16.5%	3.4%
Outpatient visits (in thousands)	198,778	269,129	285,712	43.7%	6.2%

*Percent changes are based on actual figures, not rounded.
Source: Reprinted from *Hospital Statistics*, 1990–1991 edition, by American Hospital Association, p. xxxii, with permission of American Hospital Association, © 1991.

Hospitals can also be classified by religious affiliation. Catholic hospitals, represented by the Catholic Health Association (CHA), are a major segment of the religious hospital group. In the United States there are 613 Catholic hospitals accounting for 157,133 beds.[4]

GROWTH IN THE HOSPITAL INDUSTRY

During the past decade, hospitals have been forced to adapt to changes in the economy, technology, and delivery of health care services. As a result, the number of hospitals has declined since 1980. Some hospitals have closed, others have merged and still others have become nursing homes or providers of other hospital services. There are fewer rural hospitals today than a decade ago, and there has been a decline in the number of hospital beds as well. The average length of stay for patients and the number of admissions has also declined. For the most part, these decreases are a reflection of improvements in medical technology and hospital reimbursement systems.

WHAT KIND OF SERVICES DOES THE HOSPITAL INDUSTRY PROVIDE?

Though there has been a decline in the nation's hospital-bed capacity over the past decade, hospitals now provide increased services on an outpatient basis (Figure 2-1). The movement toward outpatient care is a result of extraordinary technological advancements and increased hospital efficiency in the delivery of patient care. In 1984, about 50 percent of community hospitals provided outpatient care, whereas today, almost all community hospitals have outpatient departments. Many community hospitals also provide ambulatory surgery services. Today, three times as many hospitals as in 1978 offer medical rehabilitation services on an outpatient basis. About one-fifth of hospitals treat patients with alcohol and drug abuse problems as outpatients. Nearly all (94 percent) of community hospitals have 24-hour staffed emergency departments, though there has been a decrease in the number of hospitals offering trauma care centers, largely due to the high operating costs of such units.[5] As the 65 and older population continues to grow, hospitals have expanded their long-term care services (74 percent in the past eight years) and created skilled nursing facilities (SNFs).[6] Today, 34 percent of community hospitals also provide home care services as compared to only 11 percent in 1980 (Table 2-2).[7]

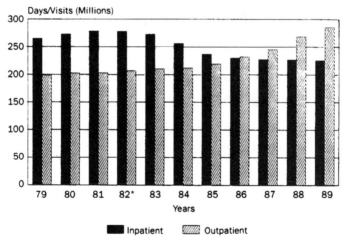

*Outpatient visit data for 1982 has been estimated using statistical techniques in order to compensate for a change in the reporting method for outpatient visits in 1982.

Figure 2-1 Community Hospital Inpatient Days vs. Outpatient Visits. *Source:* Reprinted from *Hospital Statistics,* 1990–1991 edition, by American Hospital Association, p. xxxvii, with permission of American Hospital Association, © 1991.

Table 2-2 Trends in Selected Services of Community Hospitals, 1984 and 1988-89 (Number/Percentage of Reporting Hospitals with Selected Service)

	1984		1988		1989	
	Number of Hospitals	Percent	Number of Hospitals	Percent	Number of Hospitals	Percent
Ambulatory surgery	4,836	90.7	4,989	95.1	4,886	95.2
Birthing rooms	2,449	45.9	3.322	63.3	3,351	65.3
Blood bank	3,923	73.6	3,675	70.1	3,589	69.9
Emergency department	5,064	95.0	4,935	94.1	4,846	94.4
Outpatient alcoholism/chemical dependency	767	14.4	990	18.9	1,037	20.2
Physical therapy	4,830	90.6	4,486	85.5	4,338	84.5
Trauma care	938	17.6	703	13.4	629	12.3
Volunteer services	3,712	69.6	3.477	66.3	3,427	66.8
Outpatient rehabilitation	1,939	36.4	2,408	45.9	2,501	48.7
Outpatient department	2,634	49.4	4,064	77.5	4,153	80.9
Home health care	1,167	21.9	1,809	34.5	1,784	34.7
Hospice	578	10.8	767	14.6	804	15.7
Number of hospitals reporting	5,331		5,244		5,134	

Source: Reprinted from *Hospital Statistics,* 1990–1991 edition, by American Hospital Association, pp. xxxix, with permission of American Hospital Association, © 1991.

WHAT ABOUT HOSPITAL FINANCES?

Expenditures in community hospitals totaled 168 billion dollars in 1988.[8] Labor expenditures, including payroll expenses and employee benefits, account for more than one-half of community hospitals' total expenditures. Medical supplies, pharmaceuticals, food, utilities and housekeeping, and administrative supplies make up another third. However, capital expenses for the hospital industry are approximately 15 billion dollars per year or 9 percent of the total expenses.[9] Many hospital physical plants were constructed just following World War II. These buildings need continuous repairs as they age, placing increasing pressure on the hospital industry's need for additional capital financing (Figure 2-2).

Approximately one-half of community hospitals' gross revenues come from Medicare and Medicaid. About one-third is generated from other third-party payers, such as private insurance companies. Only a small percentage of revenues

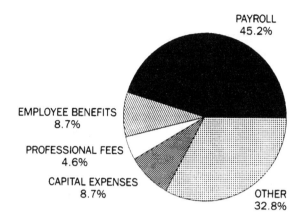

Figure 2-2 Community Hospital Expenditures, 1989. *Source:* Reprinted from *Hospital Statistics,* 1990–1991 edition, by American Hospital Association, p. xxxv, with permission of American Hospital Association, © 1991.

comes from patients who pay themselves (Figure 2-3). Since 1982, growth in revenues has been reduced to an annual rate of 10 percent.[10]

Many hospitals are facing increased financial difficulty. In 1988, 65 percent of hospitals lost money on patient care services.[11] Hospitals also suffer losses due to bad debts and charity care.

Other factors contributing to the rise in hospital expenditures are expensive technological changes in medical care and equipment, increased patient demand,

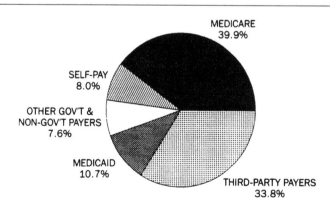

Figure 2-3 Community Hospital Gross Patient Revenue By Payer Source, 1989. *Source: Reprinted from* Hospital Statistics, 1990–1991 edition, by American Hospital Association, p. xxxv, with permission of American Hospital Association, © 1991.

and the rising cost of labor and supplies. Most other industries have increased their output by combining improvements in the organization of productive activity with the substitution of capital equipment for labor. However, the hospital industry is a highly intensive labor industry; the substitution of capital equipment for labor is not readily accomplished. Indeed, improvements in medical technology have frequently led to changes not only in the types of cases treated by hospitals but also in methods of treatment that frequently require both more expensive equipment and more highly skilled and technical labor. The public continues to use more health services. This increased use is primarily in the outpatient areas. During the last several years, hospital admissions which had increased during the 1970s began to decrease. Hospital occupancy rates also declined. However, outpatient visit to hospitals increased 85 percent between 1970–1987. Today, many complex diagnostic and therapeutic procedures are done on an outpatient basis.[12]

NOTES

1. *Hospital Statistics, 1989–1991 Ed.,* (Chicago, Ill.: American Hospital Association).

2. Ibid.

3. Ibid.

4. Source: Catholic Health Association of the United States, 4455 Woodson Road, St. Louis, MO 63134.

5. *Hospital Statistics 1989–91 Ed.,* (Chicago, Ill.: American Hospital Association).

6. Ibid.

7. Ibid.

8. Ibid.

9. Ibid.

10. Ibid.

11. Ibid.

12. Ibid.

Part II

Managing the Hospital

Chapter 3

Organization

Key Terms

Classical theory of organization • Bureaucratic organization • Span of control • Chain of command • Specialization • Pyramid organization • Matrix organization • Product line management • Line and staff—the organization chart • Chief executive officer • A team of three • Power • Corporate restructuring • Parent holding company • Multihospital system • Alliances

---

INTRODUCTION

There are two fundamental ways to view a hospital organization. One may look at the overview, or one may consider the departmental organization. Most hospitals in the United States tend to be traditionally organized, that is, they tend to follow the classical theory of organization. The traditional organization structure derives from the theory of bureaucracy described by the nineteenth-century German sociologist Max Weber (1864–1920).

Hospitals are mainly bureaucratic organizations and use bureaucratic principles. A principle of bureaucratic organization that applies effectively to hospitals is the grouping of individual positions and clusters of positions into a hierarchy or pyramid. Another effective principle of hospital organization is the consistent system of rules. Hospital rules are really guidelines or official boundaries for actions within the hospital. Examples of such rules include the set of personnel policies outlined in the personnel handbook or written nursing procedures for the care of patients in each nursing unit. Hospitals also use the principle of span of control very effectively. Under the concept of span of control, there is a limit to the number of persons a manager can effectively supervise. In a hospital a span of control of between five and ten people in a given functional area is normal to achieve operational effectiveness. This is especially true in classical functional areas such as housekeeping, dietary, and nursing. There is the division and specialization of labor in hospitals also. Specialization refers to the ways a hospital organizes to identify specific tasks and assign a job description to each person. For example, a nurse's aide has a specific task to perform that is different from that of a physician, a registered nurse, or a medical technologist.

HOW HOSPITALS ARE ORGANIZED

The most popular and traditional hospital structure is a pyramid or hierarchical form of organization. In this arrangement, individuals at the top of the pyramid (e.g., department heads) have a specified range of authority, and this authority is passed down to employees at the lower levels of the pyramid in a chain-of-command fashion (Figure 3-1). In this way, hospital authority is dispersed throughout

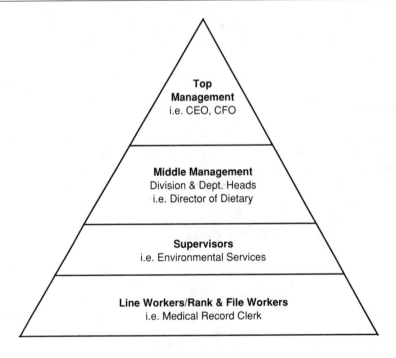

Figure 3-1 Pyramid Organization. *Source:* Author.

the organization. Hospitals encourage a pyramid type structure, with supervisors delegating to two or three subordinates who in turn delegate further down the pyramid.

A second type of organizational scheme is a matrix organization, whereby the hospital organization operates more horizontally than vertically (Figure 3-2). This arrangement is oriented to solving problems or managing projects, and the authority within a give project rests with a designated project manager rather than with the chief executive officer or department manager.

Finally, there is a hybrid organizational arrangement known as product line management. Under this scheme, hospitals or divisions within hospitals are organized according to product line categories. These categories may be referred to as strategic business units. For example, a hospital might select to organize around its surgical or obstetrical services called products, rather than around formal departments such as nursing.

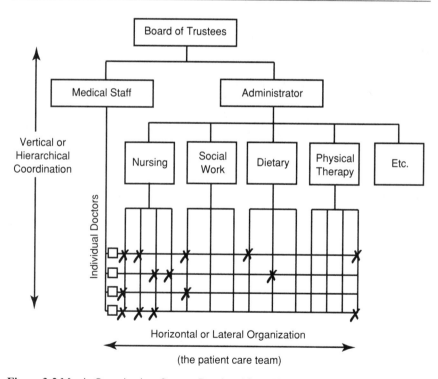

Figure 3-2 Matrix Organization. *Source:* Reprinted from *Hospital Administration*, Vol. 17, No. 4, p. 20, with permission of the Foundation of the American College of Healthcare Executives, © 1972.

LINE AND STAFF FUNCTIONS

Another important principle of organization that works well in the hospital is the differentiation between line and staff work. Perhaps the best way to view the difference between line and staff is to regard the line authority in the hospital as connoting direct supervision over subordinates (e.g., the head nurse is directly responsible for the work of the employees under that position's supervision). The delineation between line and staff is very noticeable in the nursing services department; the line authority is carried out by managers (that is, directors, assistant directors, supervisors, and head nurses), and the educational component (inservice nursing) is an advisory or staff function that supports the line authority.

THE ORGANIZATION CHART

In a typical Hospital Organization Chart (Figure 3-3), the governing body of the organization is generally referred to as the board of governors, board of trustees, or board of directors. The board delegates authority to the chief executive officer (CEO) who may have the title director, administrator or president of the hospital. (At a later point we will examine the various titles of the chief executive officer). The CEO usually has some flexibility in structuring the administration of the hospital, as shown in the lower half of the organization chart (Figure 3.3). But again, the same general administrative hierarchical principles apply. The administrator generally has associate administrators, assistant administrators, or administrative assistants to handle the various organizational and operational aspects of the day-to-day functioning of the hospital. It is usual for a CEO to have support from a vice president, chief operating officer (COO), or various other assistant administrators. The number of such executive vice presidents will vary by hospital size. It is common for hospitals in the 200–300 bed range to have one or two assistant administrators. Generally, this number tends to increase proportionately to the number of beds in the hospital. The organization chart illustrates how the span of control for the CEO and the vice presidents follows the span-of-control principle in the classical organization theory.

Following the vice president level in the hospital organization chart is the middle management group. This represents the departmental level of management. In the departmental or functional organization of the hospital, there are generally at least four major types of functions to be carried out: (1) the nursing functions, (2) the business or fiscal functions, (3) the ancillary or professional services, and (4) the support services. It is usual for a hospital to have under the CEO at least four distinctive administrative or functional groupings with a manager responsible for each of these areas. Frequently, at this stage of the game,

CEO's and managers start drawing neat little boxes on their organization charts, as was done in Figure 3.3.

Although an organization chart serves a purpose, in many instances it also has severe limitations. One of the limitations is that it does not show the hospital's informal organization. Also, physicians and other members of the medical staff are not generally shown in any strict formal authority relationships on most organization charts. Though many of the resources of the hospital are often available to the physician in order to meet the physician's and patient's needs, hospitals have not been able to show effectively the resulting relationships on most organizational charts.

A TEAM OF THREE

One of the reasons that hospitals are so complex lies in the relationships between the three major sources of power: the board, the CEO or management, and the hospital's medical staff. These relationships may be regarded as a kind of three-legged stool or a tripartite hospital governance concept. Just as the activities of the medical staff impact significantly on the management and governance of the institution, so does the board's action impinge on the doctors. The main organizational units that enable the medical staff to relate formally to the board are the medical staff's executive committee and the board's joint conference committee. However, the more dynamic links between the board and the medical staff are in the informal day-to-day dealings between the two groups, both in the hospital setting and socially outside the institution. Also, many hospitals have found it beneficial to have one or perhaps two physicians serve as voting members on the board. Thus, there is a team approach to hospital organization.

POWER

It is dangerous to generalize about power relationships in American hospitals. Historically, hospital power has rested somewhere between the board of directors, the management, and the physicians or medical staff. One observer notes that the power of the administrator appears to be increasing with respect to both trustee groups and the medical staff.[1] The point is that many of the physicians on the medical staff are present (in the hospital) part time, whereas the CEO and the management team have full-time hospital responsibilities. Furthermore, there are more physicians employed in and using the hospital today than ever before, and the physicians' impact is gaining importance. Their presence is integral to both the hospital and the organization of the hospital. In equal measure, because U.S. Courts have decided that boards of trustees have ultimate responsibilities, particularly in quality assurance, the board's importance is also growing. A board's fi-

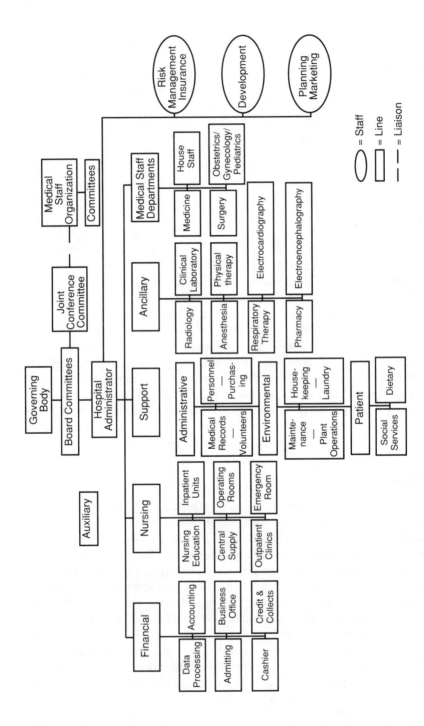

Figure 3-3 A Typical Hospital Organization Chart

duciary responsibilities as mandated by the courts have thus brought the trustees into greater involvement with the hospital and given them a greater stake in the power of the institution.

CORPORATE RESTRUCTURING IN THE HOSPITAL

Corporate restructuring or the segmentation of certain hospital assets and functions into separate corporations has become a popular strategy for hospitals to assist them in adapting to changes in regulations and reimbursement. The most common form of corporate restructuring is when a hospital becomes a subsidiary of a parent holding company or foundation (Figure 3-4). Inpatient care usually remains as the primary function of the hospital corporation, and non-provider functions may be transferred to other corporations related to the hospital. The parent holding company and non-hospital subsidiaries are able to enter into less restrictive joint ventures with physician groups and other health care providers than allowed by the traditional hospital structure. The traditional reasons for corporate restructuring include the optimization of third-party reimbursement, tax considerations, government regulation, flexibility, and diversification.

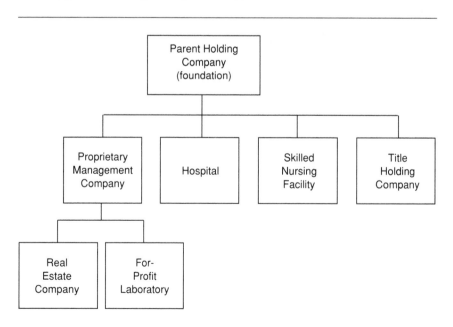

Figure 3-4 Hospital Restructuring. *Source:* Reprinted from *A Layman's Guide to Hospitals III: Hospital Corporate Reorganizations* by Coopers & Lybrand with permission of Coopers & Lybrand, © 1981.

MULTIHOSPITAL SYSTEMS

An increasing number of freestanding hospitals are becoming part of a large multihospital system. A multihospital system is two or more hospitals that are managed, leased, or owned by a single institution. Some of the common advantages of multihospital systems include economics of scale with management and purchasing, the ability to provide a wide spectrum of care, and increased access to capital markets.

Another development among nonprofit hospitals has been the creation of alliances. An alliance is a formal arrangement among several hospitals and/or hospital systems that functions according to written rules. Unlike hospitals within a multihospital system, those in an alliance retain their autonomy. The advantage of an alliance is the development of a network of support among hospitals. For example, hospitals might join together in an alliance to gain purchasing power or form a preferred provider organization to offer selected services to customers or patients at special rates.

NOTE

1. W. Richard Scott, "The Medical Staff and the Hospital: An Organizational Perspective," *The Hospital Medical Staff*, November 1973, p. 35.

The Governing Body

INTRODUCTION

The governing body of a voluntary (not-for-profit) hospital, also referred to as the board of trustees, board of directors, or board of governors, is the organized entity with ultimate responsibility for all decisions. The board essentially functions as the hospital owners and is accountable to the community.

The governing body is responsible for the medical staff's actions, and it hires the administrator. Trustees undertake the ultimate responsibilities of managing the assets of the hospital and of setting policy; they assume a fiduciary responsibility. The courts have found that the governing body has to be responsible for all activities within the hospital. Members who serve on the governing body thus clearly have a very weighty responsibility.

Trustees are private citizens who simply want to help their neighbors and community. One of the original reasons for establishing private citizens as hospital trustees was to secure financial support for the institution. By appointing local citizens who had some influence and affluence, the hospital could guarantee a certain amount of contributions to underwrite the care of the poor and the hospital's overall operation. In years past, hospital boards were often appointed so that the hospitals could obtain monetary benefits from their members. Now hospital boards frequently appoint individuals who have particular skills that can help the hospital, for example, with legal advice, accounting assistance, or business and management support. Today's hospital has a host of legal and accreditation requirements. It is the board of trustees that is required by law to watch over the hospital and its operations.

Hospital trustees generally serve without pay; they are prohibited from profiting financially from their membership on the board of trustees. The rewards for being a trustee are the satisfaction of having rendered a service to others in the community and the receipt of some measure of community status by being on the board. Because the trustees represent the ownership of the hospital, they have the ordinary liability of any owners of property. But they have the additional burden of protecting the patients from all foreseeable and preventable harm.

Since Watergate there has been an increased sensitivity to conflicts of interest in our American institutions. As part of a public service establishment, hospital trustees may be vulnerable in matters involving a conflict of interest. Hospitals are coming increasingly under public scrutiny. Some areas, including New York City and Washington, D.C., have prohibited hospital trustees from directly or indirectly doing business with the hospitals in which they serve. More commonly, a state will require that trustees make full public disclosure of their business interests and dealings with the hospitals they represent. Hospitals are well-advised to comply to the fullest with the procedures for disclosing conflicts of interest, even though it can be shown in many cases that overlapping trustee interests can actually work to the hospital's benefit, as for example when a trustee gives an institution a favorable loan or expert advice on investments.

A PROFILE OF THE GOVERNING BODY

Just as hospitals vary considerably in size, purpose, and make-up, so do their boards. The average hospital board today has 17 members, the smaller boards may have eight or nine members, and the larger boards have around 25 members. Typically, the board's composition is dominated by business executives but also may include members of the legal and accounting professions. Physicians often serve with no voting power but as representatives of the medical staff. Interest and commitment to the hospital followed by financial business skills are the leading criteria for selecting trustees. Trustees are frequently chosen from among the more prominent members of the community. It is not uncommon to find representatives of well-established families with inherited wealth serving on boards. A more recent trend, however, has been one of providing community or consumer representation on boards. Yet, for the most part, the traditional character of the board still holds. With regard to the age of a typical board member, over 55 percent fall between the ages of 51 and 70, and 38 percent between the ages of 31 and 50.[1] The majority of board members have a business or health care background. Some 87 percent of the hospitals have CEOs as board members,[2] but only 36 percent have granted the CEO voting privileges.[3] Board membership is predominantly male, although across the United States only 8.3 percent of boards are exclusively male.[4]

Potential trustee qualifications must be carefully reviewed. Hospital trusteeship demands certain essential traits including dedication to the hospital business, management skills, involvement in the community, political influence in the community, and a cooperative and easygoing attitude.

Religiously affiliated hospitals, both Protestant and Catholic, usually have hospital boards dominated by religious individuals. Many Catholic hospitals have what might be considered internal governing boards similar to industrial corporations on which the majority of members are sisters. Some time ago, the boards of Protestant hospitals began to include external members of the lay, and today have fairly liberal governance. In recent times, many Catholic hospital boards have also been changing; many Catholic hospitals now include lay community leaders as board members.

Hospital boards typically meet between 10 and 12 times a year, usually on a monthly basis. This is reasonable considering a board may not meet during one of the summer months or during the Christmas season. Board terms vary considerably, but the average term of membership is slightly in excess of three years, with a majority of hospitals stipulating no limit on the number of consecutive terms a board member may serve.

FUNCTIONS OF THE BOARD OF TRUSTEES

The basic function of the governing body is to guide, protect, and change the hospital's service mission in accordance with the institution's structure and the needs of the community. Since the board of trustees has an explicit or implicit obligation to act on behalf of the community's interest, it has a fiduciary responsibility to the community. This responsibility is founded upon trust and confidence. It involves: (1) the formal and legal responsibility for controlling the hospital and assuring the community that the hospital works properly, (2) the responsibility to see that the hospital gains support from its community, and (3) the responsibility of ensuring that the board of trustees is accountable to the citizens and the community it serves.

Specifically, hospital trustees set hospital policies. These policies are general written statements or understandings that guide or channel the thinking and action of the medical staff and the administrator in decision making. Table 4-1 highlights the essential functions of the governing body.

Lastly, it is necessary to note specifically the role of the trustee in a hospital that is part of a multihospital system. In spite of growing centralization, hospital management usually includes some degree of dual reporting responsibility, first to the

Table 4-1 Primary Functions of the Board of Trustees

Function	Description	Example
Developing and maintaining a meaningful mission statement.	Defining the hospital's reason for being, and a recommended course of action to fulfill that mission, are among the most important contributions a board can make.	Assure access to care. Assumed obligation to provide high quality health services. Board and management active in the community.
Provide for financial stability.	The board is responsible for the financial management of the hospital; it reviews the effects of policies and programs on finances, income sources, and investments, as well as the effect on the hospital of third-party payment practices. The board also is responsible for protection of hospital assets by appropriate maintenance, security measures, bonding, and appropriate property liability insurance programs.	Invest cash balances and approve budgets. Review hospital rate structure. Plan development program and engage in fundraising.
Select and evaluate CEO.	The board selects the CEO, defines his/her responsibilities, and annually evaluates his/her performance.	Identify selection criteria. Conduct formal performance review.
Develop, maintain and monitor the long-range strategic plan.	The board ensures the existence of a plan and appropriate updating. The plan indicates the goals, policies, and programs of the hospital to meet community needs. The long-range plan examines trends in medical care and diseases as well as community demographics.	Make current decisions in line with the long-range plan. Evaluate trends in medical care and delivery. Identify services to be offered and those not to be offered.
Approve selection of medical staff and its organization.	The board is responsible for a properly functioning medical staff. The board approves medical staff appointments, privileges, and bylaws. It also approves standards set by the	Approve addition of surgeon to medical staff. Award privileges to physicians. Approve recommended reappointments. Approve utilization reports.

continues

Function	Description	Example
	medical staff, requests support information for recommendations, and takes disciplinary action.	
Ensuring high-quality care.	The board ensures the processes established in the hospital to ensure quality is being rigorously adhered to, and that the information generated by these processes results in positive patient care.	Establish accountability system to protect patients. Approve reappointments to the medical staff.
Establish board procedures for conducting business.	The board develops and follows procedures for conducting board meetings; these should be spelled out in the hospital bylaws.	Follow parliamentary procedures. Hold regular meetings. Keep minutes of meetings. Establish committee structure.
Evaluate all phases of hospital performance.	The board is responsible for knowing areas in which standards are important (including both operation of the hospital and quality of medical care), and it ensures that established standards are met.	Approve ranges for efficient departmental operation. Question high rate of normal tissues removed. Ensure compliance with various codes and standards.
Ensure hospital is meeting community health needs and that community is informed.	The board must assess community needs and must seek solutions to community health problems through the offering of appropriate services. It must keep the community informed of available services, long-range plans, and hospital rate structures.	Survey community health care needs. Provide for special health needs of the hospital's community. Represent varied community groups.

Source: Adapted from *The Guide to Governance for Hospital Trustees,* by M. Totten, J.E. Orlikoff and C. Ewell, pp. 24–33, with permission of American Hospital Association, © 1990.

local board of trustees, then to the corporate staff of the multihospital system. However, the local governing body still retains primary responsibility for key medical staff relationships. The assumption of a role as a trustee in a multihospital system need not mean the loss of autonomy of the local hospital governing board.

SELECTION AND EVALUATION OF THE CHIEF EXECUTIVE OFFICER

To assist the board of trustees in managing the hospital, the trustees have an obligation to hire a competent chief executive officer to oversee the day-to-day management of the hospital. One of the board's most important functions is the investigation, review, and selection of the CEO. Hospitals are big business, and trustees must seek executives who have strengths in planning, organizing, and controlling, as well as proven leadership skills. The board then delegates to the CEO the authority and responsibility to manage the day-to-day operations of the hospital while still retaining the ultimate responsibility for everything that happens in the hospital. Thus, the relationship between the CEO and the governing board is primarily that of employee-employer, but not in the usual sense of the term. Since the hospital is a very special type of organization, the relationship between the CEO and the governing board is in fact similar to a partnership. But just as it is the responsibility of the governing board to hire the CEO, it is also their responsibility to discharge the CEO, if necessary.

RELATIONSHIP WITH THE MEDICAL STAFF

The hospital medical staff operates under its own bylaws, rules, and regulations, but the physicians on the medical staff are accountable to the board of trustees for the professional care of their patients. The board of trustees is responsible for exercising due care in appointment of physicians to the staff. A physician's application file, including credentials and privileges requested, is carefully reviewed by the medical staff. Then, the medical staff recommends to the board of trustees which privileges the applicant should be granted. The trustees act upon these recommendations. The board could choose to grant privileges, to request further information from the medical staff, or to reject the privileges outright.

The board of trustees is legally responsible for the care rendered in the hospital by the attending physicians and hospital employees. The courts indicated in Darling v. Charleston Community Memorial Hospital that the board of trustees has a duty that may go beyond simple delegation of authority to the medical staff. In the Darling case, the court held that the hospital corporation was liable because it did not intervene, through its employees, to prevent damage that occurred to a patient through the negligence of one of the hospital's physicians.[5] In another landmark case in 1973, the courts found in the case of Gonzales v. Mercy General Hospital in Sacramento, California, and John J. Nork, M.D., that a hospital owes the patient a duty of care.[6] In this case, Dr. Nork performed 36 unnecessary operations over a nine-year period. The court noted that the board of trustees has an obligation to purge the hospital of inadequate physicians. This case reconfirmed the board's corporate responsibility for quality. It cannot be delegated.

The CEO and the chief or president of the medical staff have a major role to play also. Together with the board, they develop and implement a quality assurance program. The board's job is to monitor the program. This includes receiving monthly reports on the medical staff's performance as measured against standards; concurring with medical staff recommendations or developing the board's own recommendations to improve quality in the institution.

Boards of trustees generally delegate the day-to-day medical affairs of the hospital to the medical staff. The medical staff carries out these functions according to its own bylaws and regulations. The board's joint conference committee has representatives from the medical staff and administration and serves as the main committee between the medical staff of the board and its administrator.

HOW DOES THE BOARD OPERATE?

The board of trustees operates under the bylaws of the hospital. The bylaws spell out how a hospital board is founded and how it operates to attain its objectives. Typical bylaws include a statement on the hospital's purpose and the responsibilities of the board. They also contain a statement of authority for the board to appoint the administrator and the medical staff. In addition, the bylaws outline how board members are appointed and for what period of time. Most bylaws indicate an elaborate committee structure. It is through these committees that the governing board usually gets its work accomplished. This committee structure is frequently established along special functional lines. There is remarkable consistency throughout the nation's hospitals in board committee structure. Perhaps the reason for this consistency is the impetus toward review of hospital bylaws and suggestions from the Joint Commission on Accreditation of Healthcare Organizations (JCAHO). The most common committee is the executive committee, which is found in more than 70 percent of hospitals. Other examples include a finance committee, a planning committee, and perhaps a committee for the building and its operations and grounds. Generally, recommendations through the separate committees affect the governance, management, and administration, as well as the medical staff in the hospital.

It is the duty of the board to select carefully the members of these board committees. The caliber of the recommendations that emerge from these committees, and subsequently the caliber of the resulting board action, is frequently a function of the quality of selection that went into the committee assignments. The CEO, through the application of leadership skills and management delegation and in close relationship with these board committees, frequently provides the ultimate key to success in all aspects of the hospital operation.

Hospital boards are operating more and more like other corporate boards. Corporate board members are accustomed to providing an independent voice. Clearly hospital trustees are respected for their independence and their overview of the hospital. This is the result of an increasing need to make hospitals more efficient and competitive.

NOTES

1. Daniel R. Longo, et al., "Profile of Hospital Governance: A report from the nation's hospitals," *Trustee*, May 1990, p. 7.

2. Howard J. Anderson, "Changes in board composition, size are occurring very slowly," *Modern Healthcare*, January 1987, p. 30.

3. Ibid, p. 33.

4. Richard D. Grifford, "Are hospital boards turning corporate?" *Trustee*, August 1987, p. 11.

5. Darling v. Charles Community Memorial Hospital, 211 N.E. 2d (1965) cert. denied 383 V.S. 946 (1966).

6. Robert M. Cunningham, Jr., Governing Hospitals: Trustees and the New Accountabilities (Chicago, Ill.: American Hospital Association, 1976), p. 80.

Chapter 5

The Chief Executive Officer

Key Terms

Chief Executive Officer (CEO) • American College of Health Care Executives (ACHE) • Inside activities • Respondent superior • Outside activities • Ex officio member • Networking • Chief Operating Officer (COO)

INTRODUCTION

At one time, the Chief Executive Officer (CEO), also referred to as a hospital administrator, was likely to be chosen from the ranks of the nursing department. In many church-related hospitals, it was common for the CEO to be selected from the ranks of the religious order or from among retired clergy. These administrators were hardworking and dedicated to patient care, but they were also often trained to follow the physicians' wishes. On the other hand, some administrators, including some of the best qualified the author has known, worked their way up through the business office ranks to become the hospital's CEO. It was also common in some hospitals to have a retired businessman or physician assume the CEO position.

Such upward vertical mobility is not common today. CEOs are now products of the university. The first university course for hospital administrators started in the mid-1930s. As the field of hospital administration became more and more complex following World War II, the demand for trained hospital administrators multiplied. One of the greatest influences on the advancement of hospital administration was the formation of the American College of Health Care Executives (ACHE) in 1933. The college encourages high standards of education and ethics, and only those administrators who meet the college's requirements are admitted as members. Today, formal training of hospital administrators is provided by a number of universities in the United States and Canada. These universities offer graduate and undergraduate degrees in hospital or health care administration.

The master's degree is most widely accepted as the required academic preparation for health administration. Many programs offer a masters of business administration (MBA) while some offer the masters of public administration (MPA) or masters of public health degrees. The formal training program for hospital administrators covers three general areas: (1) administrative theory, (2) the study of various components of health care services and medical care, and (3) the study of hospital functions, including the organization and management within the hospital and the role of the hospital in the larger picture of health care delivery systems. The three basic types of skills developed in training are technical, social, and conceptual.

FUNCTIONS OF THE ADMINISTRATOR

The hospital CEO of the 1930s and 1940s dealt primarily with the internal operations of the hospital. The administrator was concerned with matters that directly affected the patients treated at the hospital. This involved bargaining with employees, developing proper benefit packages, and determining the best methods and techniques to manage the institution. However, in the 1950s and into the 1960s and 1970s, increasingly strong labor unions, third-party payers, and governmental agencies all began to impact significantly on the hospital industry. During this period, the role of the administrator became a dual one, dealing with both the inside and outside aspects of hospital management. More sophisticated and specialized management was required to operate a hospital effectively, and the CEO became more involved in activities outside the hospital.

Today the CEO has to strike the proper balance between outside and inside activities. But the main role of the CEO is to coordinate the facilities of the hospital with its resources so as to allow the medical care mission of the institution to be most efficiently and effectively carried out. Since hospitals are also businesses, their services are capable of being measured by business yardsticks. The CEO's responsibility is to handle and manage the tangibles of money, personnel, and materials. In the view of the ACHE, the responsibility of the governing body or the board of trustees is to function in a judgmental or deliberative fashion. According to the ACHE, "The governing authority appoints a chief executive responsible for the performance of all functions of the institution and accountable to the governing authority. The chief executive, as the head of the organization, is responsible for all functions including a medical staff, nursing division, technical division, and general services division which will be necessary to assure the quality of patient care."

Inside Activities

Inside activities include duties such as the review and establishment of hospital procedures, supervision of hospital employees, and operations including fiscal activities, and the maintenance of internal relations. Traditionally, it has been the CEO's job to attend to those tasks in the hospital that directly affect the patients' well-being. For example, it is the responsibility of the CEO to see that the building and its facilities are in adequate order and that the personnel are qualified to fill their specific job requirements. Legally, the CEO must answer for the acts of employees under the principle of respondent superior. Another traditional CEO function, which is even more important today, is to deal with the staff physicians. The administrator must keep both the physicians and the governing board informed about the hospital and its plans. Other important tasks involve the recruitment of new medical staff and the retention of existing staff.

Generally, CEOs attend board meetings in order to communicate ideas, thoughts, and policies that will help the hospital. They prepare and defend annual budgets to be approved by the board of trustees. This includes identifying new services that need to be offered as well as new equipment which needs to be purchased. Negotiating reimbursement rates with third-party insurance plans (such as Blue Cross and Medicare) and preparing monthly financial statements and statistical data to present to the board are among the internal tasks performed by the chief executive officer.

Maintaining a positive relationship and effective communication with the hospital's governing body, medical staff, employees, and patients is very important. The official relationship between the CEO and governing body is that of an employer and employee, but actually the CEO and the board function more as partners. The administrator is the representative of the board in the daily activities of the institution and must turn the board's power into administrative action. Indeed, the partnership relationship between the board and the administrator has been solidified now that the CEO is a voting member on many hospital governing boards. This is quite common in other industries where the CEO is also a member of the board of directors and is an equal among equals, not just an employee. Typically, when administrators are members of boards, they have the title of president of the institution working under the chairman of the board. CEOs can become active, with voting privileges, or act as ex officio members on key board committees, including the nominating, bylaws, and planning committees. However, the CEO should not be chairman of the board. The trustees on the board are stewards for the community, and the nature of this stewardship should not permit the administrator, an employee of the hospital, to be the chairman.

The CEO should act in partnership not only with the board of trustees, but also with the physicians and other health care personnel in the institution. Under the best circumstances, the administrator has a mutual understanding with, respect for, and trust in the members of the medical staff. One of the key responsibilities of the chief executive officer is to communicate with the hospital's medical staff. It is the CEO's job to see that the physicians have the proper tools in the right place at the right time in order for them to carry out their role in the hospital.

Successful CEOs must be effective in keeping their medical staff informed about organizational changes, board policies, and decisions that affect them and their patients. Hospital medical staffs, though ultimately answerable to the board and its management, are also self-governing and have their own bylaws. The administrator should be sensitive to the medical staff's needs for self-governance and support that need. From time to time, natural tensions will arise between the medical staff and the administration. Frequently the sources of this conflict can be attributed to poor communication. The CEO must communicate effectively with the medical staff if the hospital is to function efficiently. Consequently, the CEO must always be available to medical personnel.

The employee group provides many of the CEO's day-to-day challenges. The employees must look to the CEO as their work leader. It is the CEO's role to keep the employees informed of the critical role their services play in the successful operation of the hospital. This is easier to achieve with nurses and others who deliver direct patient care, but the CEO must continually be informing all employees of their mission and importance. In dealing with employees at all levels, it is critical that the CEO show objectivity, understanding, and fairness. The CEO must handle the authority to employ, direct, discipline, and dismiss employees with these important principles in mind.

Lastly, the CEO has a vital role in patient relations. The CEO must fulfill all legitimate patient requests for general comfort and care in order to assist their recovery. In dealing with patients, the CEO must also understand the needs of the patients' friends and relatives. Also, it is important that the CEO safeguard confidential patient information.

Outside Activities

The outside activities of today's CEOs are numerous. They include relating to the community, understanding governmental relationships, and participating in educational and planning activities. One of the roles of the modern administrator is to educate the community about hospital operations and health care matters. This is usually done through various hospital publications and community lectures. It is the CEO's responsibility to present a positive image of the hospital. Public relations duties are considered key outside activities, and the CEO must promote public understanding of hospital programs through the mass media. One of the most valuable accomplishments of today's CEO is the negotiating of contracts with third-party payers (insurance companies) who pay for the patients' bills. This is a time-consuming activity requiring a combination of management and negotiation skills. With the passage of Medicare in 1966, hospitals and government became more deeply intertwined. Today's CEO must stay on top of the latest government rules and regulations concerning funding, reimbursement, and planning issues. CEOs meet with governmental reimbursement agencies, planning bodies, and politicians in order to keep up-to-date and to lobby for hospital interests. CEOs may lobby on an individual basis, with area CEOs, or as part of regional or national groups through hospital associations.

Dealing with public vendors and other health administrators and agencies is vital for the CEO. It is the CEO's job to remain in close contact with the community that sponsors the hospital or health care institution. The CEO must realize that the institution has a responsibility to the public and that the public has a right to be informed. The CEO has to maintain highest ethical principles in dealing with vendors. It is the CEO who must remember impartiality and objectivity when representing the hospital in business dealings. Neither the institution nor the administrator can accept favors, commissions, unethical rebates, or gifts from vendors in turn for doing business with a certain company.

Frequently CEOs telephone each other or meet to gain additional information on a particular topic, insight, or problem, or just to discuss institutional plans and situations. This is a professional courtesy that helps the administrators to broaden their own perspectives and strengthen their problem-solving abilities. This is referred to as networking.

ASSISTANT ADMINISTRATOR OR VICE PRESIDENT

One of the most important responsibilities of the CEO is to select and hire a competent administrative staff. It is the administrator's staff that is delegated the responsibility of seeing that the hospital is run smoothly and efficiently. The assistant administrator or vice president in charge of hospital operations, also referred to as the Chief Operating Officer (COO), assists the CEO in coordinating all hospital activities such as support, ancillary, and fiscal services. Typically, there are assistant administrators or vice presidents in charge of all major functional areas in the hospital. The administrative assistant frequently is involved in staff functions and is a junior member of the hospital's administrative team. The administrative assistant plans and participates in studies and programs that help the CEO in the hospital. Frequently, the administrative assistant is a liaison between the hospital administrator and some of the other functioning hospital departments.

THE FUTURE FOR CHIEF EXECUTIVE OFFICERS

Although hospitals are not growing in numbers, they certainly have become much more complex, and by doing so, have created a middle-management level which was not there 15 or 20 years ago. This means more management positions for health care administrators. Other changes in the health care industry are also creating new jobs. With respect to female chief executive officers the future looks bright. A review of the numbers of students who are entering graduate programs in hospital administration shows a growing number of women among the entrants. A review of the progress of recent women graduates shows that over 70 percent of them got the job of their first choice and that their starting salaries were comparable to their male counterparts.[2]

NOTES

1. American College of Hospital Administrators, *Principles of Appointment and Tenure of Chief Executive Officers* (Chicago, Ill.: American College of Hospital Administrators, 1973).
2. I. Donald Snook, Jr., *Hospital Administration Careers* (Lincolnwood, Ill.: VGM Career Horizons, 1989) p. 105.

Part III

Doorways to the Hospital

Outpatient Areas

INTRODUCTION

Hospitals have shifted an increasing volume of their patient care services to the outpatient setting. Over the past five years there has been a 32 percent growth rate in outpatient or ambulatory care visits, with outpatient visits increasing from 232.8 million in 1984 to 308.1 million in 1987.[1] In 1989, 26.4 percent of total net hospital revenue was generated from outpatient services.[2]

Some reasons attributed to the move toward outpatient care include: the demand for shorter hospital stays by medicare's prospective payment system; technological advancements that make the delivery of complicated patient care safer on an outpatient basis; the need for a low-cost alternative to inpatient care; and patient preference. As a result, we now see a multitude of medical, surgical, diagnostic, and rehabilitative services provided by hospitals on an outpatient basis.

In the outpatient setting, patients are registered rather than admitted. The registration process must capture accurate patient identification and billing data since there is no second chance to correct this information in the outpatient setting. In addition to collecting patient data, registration systems (systems manual or computerized) should determine patient eligibility for services, their insurance, generate a daily outpatient schedule, and provide outpatient reports and forms. Whether a centralized or decentralized system is more efficient in handling outpatient registration depends on local hospital circumstances.

AMBULATORY SURGERY

Ambulatory surgery is defined as surgery (generally of a minor nature) that does not require the patient to remain overnight in the hospital. Though we tend to believe that ambulatory surgery is a relatively new type of species of delivery, Thomas O'Donovan, in his description of ambulatory surgery in Ambulatory Surgical Centers, Development and Management, points out that a Dr. Nichol in 1909 described to the British Medical Association several thousand operations performance on ambulatory patients in a Scottish hospital.[3] However, it was not until the 1960s that hospitals, physicians, and third-party payers began to view ambulatory surgery as a viable and necessary alternative to inpatient care.

Ambulatory surgery may be performed in a traditional controlled hospital setting whereby patients enter and leave a unit or part of a hospital. This is commonly referred to as a short procedure unit (SPU), and the hospital's existing inpatient operating rooms are used. Surgery may also be performed on the hospital campus in a separate, distinct area designated for ambulatory surgery. This is usually called a surgicenter. Satellite surgicenters that are not located on the hospital's campus and that are independently operated are commonly called free-standing surgery centers.

CLINICS

The history of the hospital outpatient clinic parallels the development of hospitals themselves. In 1752, the Pennsylvania Hospital of Philadelphia opened the first hospital clinic. This was followed by a clinic established at the Philadelphia Dispensary in 1786 and then other sites throughout the eighteenth century. These clinics primarily served the urban poor who did not have access to private physicians at that time. Over most of the past 200 years there has been very little change in the nature of the urban hospital clinic. There are, however, wide variations in types of clinics, ranging from an array of very sophisticated, "middle-class," private physician offices to large urban teaching hospitals manned by house staffs. In urban areas, clinics continue to serve mostly the indigent and to provide medical resources for those who do not have access to private physicians.

Hospital clinics generally follow the lines of specialization within the hospital medical staff. This means that hospitals offer outpatient clinics in medicine, surgery, obstetrics, gynecology, and pediatrics, in addition to the basic services. In the more technologically advanced and tertiary teaching centers, there can be as many as 50 or 60 different specialty clinics meeting some time during each month. Due to the deficit financial nature of hospital clinics and emergency rooms, hospital controllers and administrators try to have third-party payers pick up their proper portion of the bills for indigent outpatients. Another option is the dissolution of hospital clinics through the establishment of private group practices or the sharing of services.

In an attempt to make the utilization of emergency rooms more appropriate, another species of delivery has evolved known as urgent care centers, also called urgicenters. An urgicenter provides services to nonemergency patients, whose needs are positioned between an emergency room and clinic service. Some hospitals have found it valuable to keep the urgicenter on the hospital campus as part of their emergency service.

ANCILLARY OUTPATIENT SERVICES

Due primarily to the great increase in emergency department visits and associated ambulatory visits, the hospital's supporting services—laboratory, x-ray, and physical therapy—have grown considerably and now provide a major source of support for the hospital's outpatients. When patients are referred for laboratory or x-ray studies or for physical therapy treatments, rather than being registered as clinic patients, the hospital records these patients as referred outpatients. The number of patients referred to ancillary services has been on the rise, a significant factor in the hospital's revenue picture. One study showed outpatient activity in the various ancillary service departments as follows: laboratory, 17 percent; diagnostic radiology, 47 percent; therapeutic radiology, 89 percent; nuclear medicine, 29 percent; and physical therapy, 37 percent.[4]

Freestanding imaging centers also provide the traditional services offered by hospital-based outpatient radiology services. Some of these new centers are simply already existing private radiology practices with new names.

GROUP PRACTICE

Medical group practice is defined as "the application of medical services by three or more physicians formally organized to provide medical care, consultation, diagnosis and/or treatment through the joint use of equipment and personnel and with the income from medical practice distributed in accordance with methods previously determined by members of the group." The concept of group practice in medicine began to evolve around the turn of the century. Prior to that time, physicians joined together to practice medicine, but they did not consider themselves as an organized group practice.

Groups are usually organized as single-owner groups, partnerships, professional corporations (PCs), associations, or foundations. There are subdefinitions of large physician-directed multispecialty groups. The number of group practices has almost tripled over the past 20 years. In 1988 there were 16,579 group practices as compared to 6,371 in 1969.[5] Two of the largest growing specialty groups are the emergency department groups that render services to a hospital's emergency rooms and primary care service groups that are based either in the hospital itself or in the hospital's medical office building complex.

Some of the reasons physicians join a group practice are the ease of consultation; the reduction of administrative overhead and duties involved when hiring trained clerical personnel; the opportunities for physicians to recruit newer physicians to their group; financial security and incentives for the physicians; less use of hospital facilities by the physicians; improved clinical results, especially in prenatal mortality; and the tendency to improve professional competency.

MEDICAL OFFICE BUILDINGS (MOBS)

With the changing patterns of ambulatory medicine, physicians as well as hospital management have had to rethink the conventional ways of rendering service and providing resources. In many communities, the traditional office with one physician and one nurse has been rapidly disappearing. Physicians have learned that banding together in medical office buildings, sharing overhead and, in some instances, staff and other resources such as laboratory and x-ray, has provided an efficient and economical way to practice outpatient medicine.

Hospitals also have recognized that efficient outpatient care can be rendered in a systemized well-planned medical office building. The medical office building is usually a separate building, but it could include segments of existing hospitals, such as floors, wings, or towers that have been made into medical office building suites. Medical office building concepts provide an interesting example of a winning situation where their establishment is good for the hospital, the physician, and the patient. They allow for increased efficiency in patient care on an ambulatory basis. In the circumstances when the building is on the hospital campus, the patient frequently receives a one-step service of quality care supported by the hospital medical staff. Viable medical office buildings permit physician groups to establish an excellent nucleus for the development of health maintenance organizations. A medical office building stabilizes the office location of key staff physicians who might shift their offices or their allegiance to other hospitals or other communities. Also, it gives the hospital an additional tool for physician recruitment. The presence of a viable medical office building on the hospital campus or within the hospital has been shown to increase the patient census at the hospital.

The actual organization, financial structure, and legal structure for medical office building complexes vary. There are essentially four models: (1) the hospital owns and maintains the facility; (2) the medical office building is owned by the physicians, and the hospital acts as a partner to secure loans and other financial arrangements; (3) the physicians and an outside developer own the building and lease the land from the hospital; or (4) the physicians and an outside developer own the building, and the hospital leases space from the physician-developer group. Though all four models do exist, recent studies show that over 80 percent of the medical office buildings under construction are being built by hospitals.[6]

STANDARDS OF ACCREDITATION

The Joint Commission on Accreditation of Healthcare Organizations (JCAHO) has revised its standards for Hospital-Sponsored Ambulatory Care Services in order to address such issues as the responsibility for quality of care and the safety of the environment in which care is provided (Exhibit 6-1).

Exhibit 6-1 JACHO Standards for Hospital-sponsored Ambulatory Care Services

1. Ambulatory care services, whether provided through a formally organized department/service of the hospital, other organized departments/services of the hospital, or a combination thereof, are provided safely and effectively, in accordance with the mission of the hospital and the needs of the patients served, and in a manner designed to improve the quality of care.
2. Personnel are prepared for their responsibilities in the provision of ambulatory care services through appropriate education and training programs.
3. The provision of ambulatory care services is guided by written policies and procedures.
4. The hospital implements structures, systems, policies, and procedures for safety management, life safety, equipment and management, and utilities management in all areas where ambulatory care patients are provided services.
5. A medical record is maintained for every patient who receives ambulatory care services.
6. The hospital establishes structures, systems, policies, and procedures designed to improve the quality of patient care services.
7. As part of the hospital's quality assurance program, the quality and appropriateness of patient care provided by the ambulatory care department/service are monitored and evaluated in accordance with Standard QA.3 and Required Characteristics QA.3.1 through QA.3.2.8 in the "Quality Assurance" chapter of this *Manual*.

Source: Copyright 1990 by the Joint Commission on Accreditation of Healthcare Organizations, Chicago. Reprinted with permission from Accreditation Manual for Hospitals, 1990, pp. 53–63.

MAJOR GROWTH AREAS IN THE FUTURE

The future will see an even greater shift from the inpatient hospital stay to the day or ambulatory hospital concept. With this shift, there will be continued growth in the types and prevalence of alternative or substitute programs and services traditionally rendered in the inpatient setting. Some examples of existing substitute programs include: day chemotherapy programs, rehabilitative care programs, hospice care programs, pain intervention programs, and behavioral medicine programs. Although these programs still will be offered in the hospital environment, they also will be provided in separate ambulatory clinics or medical malls.

NOTES

1. "Outpatient Care: A Nationwide Revolution," *Hospitals,* August 1990, p. 28.
2. Ibid, p. 28.
3. Thomas R. O'Donovan, ed., "Ambulatory Surgical Centers," (Rockville, Md.: Aspen Publishers, Inc., 1976), p. 4.
4. "Study Shows That Outpatient Department is Major Source of Hospital Revenue," *Hospitals, J.A.H.A.,* November 1979, p. 46.
5. "Changing Face of Hospital-Sponsored Group Practice," *Medical Staff Leader, AHA,* November 1989, p. 1.
6. Marion S. Kessler and Susan Ashby, "Hospital Landlords: Trends in Leasing Medical Office Space," *The Hospital Medical Staff,* July 1979, p. 30.

Chapter 7

The Emergency Department

Key Terms

Accident room • Emergency room • Categories of emergency care • Trauma • Rotating coverage • Voluntary coverage • Board certified emergency physician • Log of patients • Internal disaster • External disaster

---

INTRODUCTION

In the early days of hospitals, the emergency room was called an accident room, or accident ward. The accident room was the place to treat patients who had surgical problems as a result of automobile accidents, home accidents, or job-related accidents. At that time, hospital management viewed the accident room as a necessary community service but not as a glamorous hospital product. General practitioners, many specialty surgeons, obstetricians, and pediatricians had very little use for the concept of accident rooms since most of their patients were seen in their offices. Accident rooms were generally staffed by the hospital interns, who were not necessarily experienced in accident situations. Typically, there were registered nurses to support the interns. A recent medical journal described the accident room this way: "It was born in the basement and was relegated to the basement until the late 1960s."[1]

Things started to change after World War II. As medical schools and teaching hospitals began to produce superspecialties, and the general practitioner began to shrink from the medical scene, it was not long before patients discovered that they had nowhere to turn for the usual minor complaints and illnesses. The path of least resistance and the one frequently open was the hospital accident room or emergency room. The accident room soon became a walk-in medical clinic in many communities.

EMERGENCY ROOM UTILIZATION

The annual number of emergency room units in the United States exceeds 86 million. The number of patient emergency room visits is on the rise.[2] Approximately 30 percent of a hospital's admissions are through the emergency room and 50 percent of a hospital's total revenue is generated on patients who use or come through the emergency department.[3]

For a mobile population like that of the United States, the use of emergency services for family care has become a way of life. The relocation of families from one area to another has had a profound impact on the use of emergency rooms. When an illness strikes before the family has had time to select a private physician, the hospital becomes the natural place to seek care.

The move of middle-income families and their physicians to suburban areas has left urban hospitals surrounded by economically disadvantaged families who depend on the hospital for medical care. Still, patients who are financially able to pay for care sometimes choose emergency room services if they live a great distance from a physician's office. Many patients have learned that their medical needs are obtained much more quickly in hospital emergency rooms. Some patients believe that emergency rooms have better treatment facilities than physicians' offices. Emergency rooms are being used as afterhours' physicians' offices and have become 24-hour outpatient clinics. This places a heavy burden on the facilities, space, staff, and finances of the hospital.

CATEGORIZATION OF EMERGENCY FACILITIES

Not all hospitals operate emergency rooms, nor are hospitals required to do so by law, regulation, or the Joint Commission on Accreditation of Healthcare Organizations. However, if a hospital does operate an emergency service, it is held to all appropriate rules and regulations of third-party agencies. In the early 1970s, various organizations, regions, and states began to review the concept of categorizing the different emergency facilities into the levels of care that they are capable of providing. There are four categories of emergency care based on the level and depths of services. Table 7-1 illustrates the four levels of emergency services according to the JCAHO.

Trauma is the leading cause of death in Americans under 34 years of age.[4] Studies show that one-third of the trauma deaths that occur in hospitals without designated trauma units are preventable.[5] As a result, hospitals have established trauma centers. A trauma center is a high-tech center that provides emergency care

Table 7-1 Levels of Emergency Services

Level I	A Level 1 emergency department/service offers comprehensive emergency care 24 hours a day, with at least one physician experienced in emergency care on duty in the emergency care area.
Level II	A Level II emergency department/service offers emergency care 24 hours a day, with at least one physician experienced in emergency care on duty in the emergency care area, and with specialty consultation available within approximately 30 minutes by members of the medical staff or by senior-level residents.
Level III	A Level III emergency department/service offers emergency care 24 hours a day, with at least one physician available to the emergency care area within approximately 30 minutes through a medical staff call roster.
Level IV	A Level IV emergency service offers reasonable care in determining whether an emergency exists, renders lifesaving first aid, and makes appropriate referral to the nearest organizations that are capable of providing needed services.

Source: Copyright 1990 by the Joint Commission on Accreditation of Healthcare Organizations, Chicago. Reprinted with permission from *Accreditation Manual for Hospitals, 1990,* pp. 53–63.

to trauma victims, and it is usually integrated with an air transport system. There are two levels of trauma centers, with Level I treating 60–100 trauma victims annually and Level II treating 350–600 patients per year. Most trauma centers have had an adverse financial impact on hospitals due to unpaid bills and extraordinarily high operating costs. This has resulted in trauma center closings, particularly in urban hospitals.

PHYSICAL FACILITIES

It is advisable that the emergency department be located on the ground floor with easy access for patients and ambulances. Generally, it is best to have it separated from the main entrance of the hospital. The emergency department should make its entrance easily visible from the street, for example, with proper lighting and signs. It is very important that the ambulance entrance to the emergency department be large enough to admit one or more ambulances negotiating with stretchers. Emergency departments should have waiting rooms sufficient for patients and their families and friends as well as telephone areas and rest rooms close by. X-ray and laboratory services should be easily accessible to the emergency department. Over 40 percent of emergency patients require x-rays, and over 20 percent need laboratory studies. If emergency departments handle a patient volume in excess of 1,000 patients per month or handle an unusually high number of fracture cases, they may have their own x-ray facilities. A portable x-ray apparatus is seldom satisfactory. If an x-ray unit is located within the emergency room, provision must be made for the consultation services of radiology technicians and radiologists.

Generally, the emergency department has at least two or three functional areas. Typically, there is the trauma area where the severely injured surgical cases are handled. There should be a medical examining area nearby and a casting area for orthopedic problems. There should be observation beds for patients who need to stay in the emergency room area (for neurological and other medical reasons). These observation beds can be used as an interim area before the patient moves to the inpatient nursing unit. The Committee on Trauma of the American College of Surgeons has published a model of a hospital emergency department that outlines in clear, understandable detail the proper physical facilities requirements and suggests layouts for the emergency department.

ORGANIZATION

The emergency room is generally considered to be an outpatient nursing unit in the hospital organization. However, unlike other hospital nursing units, the medical staff plays a major onsite role in the emergency department and thereby complicates the organization of the emergency room. Typically, the nursing service staffs the emergency department with nursing and auxiliary personnel as they do any other nursing unit. However, since physician coverage is required in the unit there is a management partnership between physicians and nurses in this unit.

The current organizational trend in emergency services is for the unit to be a separate and distinct department under the direction of a full-time physician director. This evolution from a nursing unit within a nursing service to a physician-directed department is more prominent in the larger hospitals that employ full-time physicians to staff the activity. The physicians generally report directly to the medical staff, to the management of the hospital, or through a committee called the emergency department committee of the medical staff. The emergency department committee is frequently the committee of the medical staff that has to evaluate and plan the operations of the emergency department by enlisting the opinions and skills of a variety of concerned persons in the hospital. Typically, the emergency department committee is made up of representatives from the medical staff, nursing staff, and administration. This committee formulates the medical-administrative policies to guide the emergency room operations. It also examines the level and quality of emergency care rendered in the department. This committee may be involved in analyzing the flow of patients and the relationship of the emergency department patients to the ancillary services, such as x-ray and laboratory.

ADMISSIONS

It is important to realize that the emergency department has a significant impact on the hospital's inpatient population. As previously mentioned, about one-third of the hospital's admissions come through the emergency department. It has been noted that "not only do emergency admission patients generally remain in the hospital for a longer period of time, but also their admissions usually entail greater use of ancillary services than that which occurs with scheduled patients. Therefore, reliable gauges of the extent to which the emergency department activity is converted to inpatient hospital use are particularly important to planners, administrators, and fiscal intermediaries."[6]

Emergency department patients will follow one of five avenues after coming for service. The patient may (1) be treated and sent home; (2) be treated, held over in the emergency department for observation in the "holding rooms," and then sent home; (3) require emergency surgery, go directly to the operating room, and then to an inpatient unit; (4) be admitted directly to the inpatient unit; or (5) be stabilized in the emergency department and transferred to another hospital for admission.

PHYSICIAN COVERAGE OF THE EMERGENCY DEPARTMENT

There are a variety of methods employed to provide physician coverage for hospital emergency service. General legislation, shifts in population growth, and additional emphasis on ambulatory medicine are some of the factors to be considered when selecting the proper staffing method.

Physicians on the medical staff may be required to provide rotating coverage or the hospital may permit the attending staff to provide voluntary coverage in staffing the emergency department. The medical staff may be divided into two or more groups that voluntarily rotate and may also be used for specialty referrals from the emergency department. In large teaching hospitals, it is common for residents and medical students to staff the emergency room. A large group of private practitioners may contractually agree to staff the emergency department while retaining their individual practices. Sometimes a small group of specialty physicians may staff the emergency service under contract, and they do not maintain a private practice. Lastly, a hospital may employ full-time salaried physicians. It is important to note that contracts for emergency department coverage do give rise to legal questions and issues involving the hospital's liability for malpractice or negligency by any of the doctors.

Since 1979, when emergency medicine became recognized as a medical specialty, hospitals have been replacing their part-time staff with emergency specialists. Residency-trained emergency graduates of accredited programs are eligible for board certification. In order to become a board-certified emergency physician, the practitioners must successfully complete the examination given by the American Board of Emergency Medicine.

RECORDS

Good medical and administrative practice demands that the hospital initiate medical records on each patient visiting the emergency department. It is also necessary for the hospital to protect itself legally. Most emergency department medical records are simple compared to the extensive inpatient records. Generally, they carry administrative and basic statistical data about the patient with a place for appropriate baseline clinical data, such as blood pressure and temperature, plus a space for physicians' and nurses' notes. Generally the emergency record is limited to one sheet. If a patient is admitted to the hospital, the emergency service record accompanies the patient and is made a part of the patient's inpatient medical chart. If the patient is not admitted, the emergency record is retained in the emergency department, and another copy is sent to the medical records department for proper storage. It is common practice in many emergency departments to have several carbon copies of the medical record. As a professional courtesy, emergency personnel forward one copy to the patient's attending physician to aid in the patient's future care and provide continuity of care.

It is typical for emergency departments to maintain a register or log of patients. This is usually an appointment book or a sheet of paper containing such information as the patient's name, date of admission to the emergency department, age, sex, type of medical or surgical problem, and the disposition of the case. The emergency department log provides information for analysis and studies, such as frequency of visits, the nature of the visits, and so forth. When patients arrive at the emergency department with a previous inpatient admission history at that hospital, the physicians and nurses treating the patient will usually request the patient's prior inpatient medical record so that proper treatment can be given to the patient.

FINANCIAL IMPLICATIONS

Because the emergency department is generally open 24 hours a day, with heavy costs in the area of physician salaries and around-the-clock nursing staff, the hospital must look at the broader implications of providing emergency service. A traditional view of the emergency department is that it is a drain on hospital resources. Depending on the financial status of the outpatients visiting the department, especially in urban areas, it could be a financial drain. In an average hospital, a significant portion of inpatients come through the emergency department. Studies have shown that emergency department patients are high utilizers of ancillary services of the hospital. The high use of the ancillary services by both outpatients and inpatients contributes to the increased charge structure and hopefully improves cash flow for the hospitals.

Typically, one-third of the bill for a hospital emergency patient stems from the emergency department; the remaining charges are generated through the utilization of ancillary services. With the use of ancillary services and the element of free care in the outpatient aspect of the emergency services, the financial dimension of the emergency department is complex.

It is common for urban emergency departments to run a high level of bad debts and free care. The principal factor causing this financial drain is the emergency service's third-party insurance demographics. Because of the physician availability problem in our urban areas, a large number of welfare, Medicaid, and indigent patients use the emergency service as a substitute primary care physician. In many states, the government's Medicaid outpatient reimbursement formulas do not meet the hospital's costs, thereby leaving the emergency department with a large financial deficit and inadequate cash flow.

The typical patient's bill for a visit to the emergency department may include three different types of charges. First, there is a basic visit charge that will vary between hospitals; this is the part of the bill that helps pay for the fixed and overhead charges in the department. Second, there may be a separate charge for physicians' services. If the hospital employs the emergency department physician or the house staff is used, there will not be a separate charge for professional services. Third, there may be an ancillary or special services charge for drugs, x-rays, or laboratory work.

The emergency service must be viewed in the sense of total hospital impact rather than as a restricted departmental outpatient center. Emergency departments may increase the hospital's census and cash flow in the inpatient area. Improved physical facilities, competent professional staffing, and the image of high quality patient care in the community all seem to add up to increased volume in the hospital's emergency rooms, which then tends to lower the cost per visit.

LEGAL IMPLICATIONS

Perhaps the most common legal question arising in the emergency department is the issue of treating minors who come to the emergency department without their parents or guardian. Hospitals have to weigh the threat of assault and battery versus the matter of rendering necessary emergency care. Kucera reports the following case:

> In the landmark case of Wilmington General Hospital vs. Manlow, the
> emergency department nurse refused to admit a four-month-old infant

who was seriously ill with diarrhea. His temperature was 102 degrees. The nurse refused to admit the infant because the child's parents did not have an authorization slip from their family physician who had prescribed the medication for the child. The parents took the child home where he died later that afternoon. The Delaware Supreme Court held liability on the part of the hospital may be predicated on the refusal of service to the patient in the case of an unmistakable emergency if the patient relied upon a well established custom of the hospital to render aid in such a case.[7]

Following this landmark court decision, many states now maintain that the hospital holds itself out to the public as a provider of emergency medical services, and the hospital is accordingly under an obligation to provide emergency care to any individual who requests it. Lawyers advise emergency department physicians that if it is a threat to life and limb it is far better to treat the child even in the absence of securing parental consent than to send the minor out of the emergency department.

Another important issue in the area of hospital liability is the matter of the hospital's responsibility to inform the emergency department patient in layman's terms about the type and timing of any recommended follow-up medical care. Many hospitals, in attempting to adopt this principle, give the patient written follow-up instructions to reduce their liability and to improve communications.

The presence of intoxicated patients in the emergency department usually creates a sense of turmoil. Such patients can be loud, hostile, demanding, and difficult to deal with. Many times these patients may be escorted into the area by police, often from the scene of a recent accident. Frequently the police authorities ask for a blood alcohol test. This is a clinical laboratory procedure to determine the level of alcohol present in the patient's blood at any given time, the results of which could prove whether the patient is legally intoxicated. Hospitals must be cautious in permitting blood alcohol tests to be taken without the patient's concurrence (the patient's signed permission). Since requests for these tests may occur frequently, the emergency department staff must be thoroughly familiar with the local laws, statutes, and regulations that apply to the taking of blood alcohols.

Legally all government hospitals and, in some jurisdictions, hospitals receiving government financial support may not refuse emergency care on the basis of race, color, creed, or national origin. All hospitals participating in Medicare that have emergency departments must provide medical services to anyone needing emergency care. Patients with an unstable condition may not be transferred to another hospital without authorization from medical personnel, patient consent, and an agreement by the receiving hospital.

HANDLING DISASTERS

Hospitals should be prepared for three kinds of disasters. The first is an internal hospital disaster, such as an explosion or major fire. The second is an external disaster, such as a hurricane, tornado, flood, or transportation accident. The third is a forewarned disaster, such as the receipt of a large number of patients from a neighboring hospital that has had to evacuate.

The Joint Commission on Accreditation of Healthcare Organizations requires that hospitals have an emergency preparedness program to manage natural disasters or other emergencies that disrupt the ability to provide care and treatment. The program should include the following: a description of the hospital's role in community-wide emergency preparedness; hospital plans to implement specific procedures; provisions for managing space, supplies, communications, and security; staff responsibilities and functions; provisions for managing patients; staff emergency training; and semiannual practice drills.[8]

REFERENCES

1. Eugene J. Riley, "Emergency Evolution," *St. Josephs Hospital Bulletin,* 1977.
1A. *Hospital Statistics 1989–91 Ed.,* American Hospital Association, p. 12.
2. Ibid.
3. Ibid.
4. "Trauma in the Emergency Department," *Modern Healthcare,* April 1988, p. 30.
5. "Trauma Systems," *JAMA,* June 1988, p. 3,597.
6. Marion S. Kessler and Karen C. Wilson, "Emergency Department Key Factor in Hospital Admissions," *Hospitals, JAHA,* 16 Dec. 1978, p. 87.
7. William R. Kucera, "Narrow Definition of Emergency Can Spell Litigation," *The Hospital Medical Staff,* September 1978, p. 23.
8. The Joint Commission AMH Accreditation Manual for Hospitals (Chicago, Ill.: 1989), p. 197.

Chapter 8

The Admitting Department

Key Terms

Patient information booklets • Patient's Bill of Rights • Emergency admissions • Urgent admissions • Elective admissions • Preadmission testing • Bed allocation policy • Bedboards • General consent form

---

INTRODUCTION

Admitting is the process whereby an individual becomes a hospital inpatient. The admitting department has changed over the last decade. It once was a relatively easy matter for the patient or the patient's family to give the admissions clerk the routine factual information necessary to admit the patient. Those days are gone. A host of external factors—the legal system, third-party payers, government regulations and review programs—have changed the role of the admissions officer. Today, more and more people interact with the admissions department as an individual patient's case management has become very important to hospitals and payers under prospective payment reimbursement systems.

THE DEPARTMENT'S ROLE IN PUBLIC RELATIONS

Since the admitting department functions as an early hospital control point, it assumes a significant role in hospital public relations. Essentially, this department is responsible for forming external relationships between the hospital and patients and patients' families as well as internal relationships between the hospital and admitting physicians and their office staffs. Good communication and departmental efficiency are vital to foster healthy internal and external relationships.

As the hospital doorway for patients and their families, early and often lasting impressions begin at the admitting office. A positive image can be generated through patient information booklets or brochures that are either distributed before or upon admission of the patient. Frequently these are given to the patient's family and to visitors as well. A booklet for patients outlining the "do's" and "don'ts" of the hospital stay will make the patient's hospitalization a bit more understandable and comfortable and a bit less stressful. Several years ago, the American Hospital Association developed a Patient's Bill of Rights that explained a hospital's obligations to patients and clarified the relationships among the physician, the patient, and the hospital organization during the patient's stay. This Patient's Bill of Rights could be included in the patient information booklet. In addition, patients should find the admitting staff to be sympathetic, understanding, courteous, and professional. Also, the admitting department should be tastefully decorated and designed to provide privacy for patients and their families.

The admitting department also plays a major role in sustaining positive relations with the medical staff and hospital personnel. Indeed, all who come in contact with the department will form a reaction toward the hospital based on their experience with the admitting staff. Any negative experience that a patient encounters in the admitting department may be relayed to the physician and other hospital personnel causing unnecessary negative public relations.

FUNCTIONS OF THE ADMITTING DEPARTMENT

Besides the admitting department's role as a key public relations arm of the hospital, the department is also responsible for starting to process the patient's financial information. For example, it is involved in financial interviewing, credit arrangements, and acceptance of hospital deposits for patients without insurance. The admitting department is also involved in quality and utilization processes such as preadmission registration, preadmission testing, review of hospital admission designations, and review of length of stay. Other functions in the admitting department include assigning beds, preparing the daily census, and acting as liaison with physicians' offices.

TYPES OF ADMISSIONS

It has been common practice in hospitals to classify admissions based on the patient's needs. Emergency admissions are patients who have to be immediately admitted to the hospital for life-threatening causes. When there is not a vacant inpatient bed, emergency admissions can be housed in the hospital's emergency department's holding area. The next category of admission is urgent. These patients must be admitted within 48 hours because their life or well-being could be threatened. The least critical category for admissions is elective. These patients' lives are not immediately endangered. Their admission can be delayed.

It is common for the hospital's medical staff to be asked to review or to modify these admission definitions. Also the hospital's medical staff has an obligation to review the categories of admission and define them based on local community conditions, for example, by considering the age of the population and the services available in the hospital.

PREADMISSION

Admission of a patient can be facilitated if certain tasks are handled prior to the patient being admitted to the hospital. The preadmission process involves the admissions officer receiving pertinent personal and financial data with the patient's hospital reservation. This data can be obtained by mail or telephone days in advance of the patient's actual admission. The objective of gathering preadmission data is to expedite the processing of the patients into the hospital, thereby reducing waiting time in the admissions office or the lobby.

Preadmitting also allows for more efficient scheduling of patients into the inpatient area. To accomplish this objective, the admissions office generally sends the patient certain forms in advance to be completed and to be returned to the hospital prior to admission. The forms request the patient's name, address, certain statistical information, and details on the patient's financial insurance coverage. They also often ask if the patient has special requests, for example, a specific room accommodation or any special needs during the hospitalization.

Prior to the patient's admission, certain clinical preadmission testing is conducted on many elective patients. Third-party payers concerned with the high cost of medical care encourage this preadmission testing process. The process of preadmission clinical testing involves the patient coming to the hospital for ancillary studies, including laboratory tests, x-ray examinations, or electrocardiograms. Testing is generally done on an outpatient basis prior to the day of admission. The majority of these tests turn out to be normal, or at least what the ordering physician expected. However, if an abnormality is discovered, the test results might delay a patient's surgery or at least his course of treatment. Under these circumstances, the patient might have to remain in the hospital longer than necessary. The patient may remain an outpatient until the particular problem is handled and can then enter the hospital for surgery.

Preadmission testing has four recognized benefits for the patient, the physician, and the hospital:

1. It frequently reduces the need to postpone or cancel surgery by discovering unusual test results prior to admission.

2. It allows the hospital's busy ancillary areas (x-ray and laboratory) to distribute the workload more evenly.

3. It provides information to the physician prior to the admission and makes the physician's preoperative patient workup much easier.

4. Since the testing is done on an outpatient basis, it frequently shortens the length of the patient's hospital stay; it thereby reduces the cost to the patient and to the insurance company and also frees beds for other patients.

Preadmission testing does have some drawbacks. Sometimes the patient is too ill to go to the hospital for diagnostic studies. Obviously, preadmission will not work on emergency admissions. Some patients are unwilling or unable to leave work to go to the hospital a day or two prior to admission. Some patients find it inconvenient to travel long distances to the hospital.

The Blue Cross insurance plans of this country have been the national leaders in preadmission testing. On the other hand, the Blue Cross plans and Medicare are looking very critically at unnecessary diagnostic admission procedures. It has been common for hospitals to give patients a battery of tests—such as chest x-ray, electrocardiogram, and selected chemistry studies—prior to the patient's admission. Medicare's position on routine admission studies is that

> . . . "chest" x-rays, and other diagnostic procedures performed as part of the admitting procedure to a hospital should be specifically ordered by a physician and they should be found medically necessary for the diagnosis or treatment of the illness of the patient admitted to the hospital in order to be covered. Coverage of tests routinely performed [upon a doctor's standing orders] on admission could not, therefore, generally be considered reasonable and necessary. In addition, coverage of an admission test ordered by a physician should be questioned if it is known that the same test has been performed as part of an outpatient diagnostic workup prior to admission or in connection with a recent prior admission.[1]

One benefit of the preadmission testing program is the easing of the scheduling problems in the surgical suite. Operating room time must be scheduled in advance for patients who are admitted for elective surgery. With preadmission tests already accomplished before the patient is admitted, the operating room staff can better schedule its workload. The admitting department must work very closely with the operating room scheduler to coordinate the admission and the operating room time. Some hospitals allow the admitting department to schedule surgical time in the operating room, but this is not a common practice.

CONSENT FORMS

Frequently, the admitting department is responsible for obtaining a patient's signature on certain consent forms upon admission. Consent forms generally fall into two categories: (1) consent forms for general procedures and general treatment, and (2) special consent forms for any surgical or medical procedure. Usually the admitting officer is responsible for the general consent forms, while the physicians and other clinical members of the medical team may be involved in obtaining signatures on the special consent forms, since they require informed consent. General consent forms often cover routine procedures such as laboratory work, x-rays, or simple medical treatment. Special consent forms are involved in major or minor surgery, anesthesia, radiation therapy or certain x-ray treatments, and experimental procedures.

BED ASSIGNMENTS

Beds may be assigned to patients by patient care categories, by buildings, or by floors, depending on the institution's bed allocation policy. Traditionally, bed boards or visual display boards have been used to control and monitor the assignment of beds. In some hospitals, visual display boards are being replaced by computerized displays and are being integrated with hospital information systems. These computerized systems are the same systems used by hotels to assign beds to visitors.

NOTE

1. Medicare Bulletin, 79-34, Nov. 2, 1979, AETNA Life Insurance Company, Medicare Administration. Hospital Admission and Diagnostic Procedures which are defined as "reasonable and necessary" and therefore covered under Medicare relate to Section 1862(a)(1) of the act and Section 405-310(k) of the Medicare regulations.

Part IV

The Medical Team

The Medical Staff

INTRODUCTION

The hospital medical staff is an organized body of physicians, dentists, perhaps podiatrists, and in some instances allied health staff professionals who attend patients and participate in related clinical care duties.

The medical staff has the greatest impact on the quality and quantity of care given in the hospital. The medical staff is the heart of the hospital. Members of the medical staff have been authorized by the board of trustees to attend patients in the hospital and are accountable to the governing authority. They are accountable to the hospital for high-quality patient care through the application of ethical, clinical, and scientific procedures and practices. Though the governing body has the ultimate legal and moral responsibility for the hospital, including the quality of medical care, the board of trustees cannot practice medicine and is dependent upon the members of the medical staff to admit patients and to provide quality patient care.

The medical staff is appointed by the board of trustees. The staff is then expected to formulate its own medical policies, rules, and regulations and to be responsible to the board for the quality of patient care. Though the medical profession is a highly disciplined, professional group, it is made up of highly individualistic members who have their own unique approaches to medicine and organizational relationships. Therefore, the task of coordinating the efforts of the medical staff with the board of trustees, the administrator, and the rest of the hospital can be a challenging one.

BECOMING A PHYSICIAN

The training period to become a doctor is a long and arduous one. Three or four years of undergraduate work, heavy on courses in biology and the other sciences, is followed by the Medical College Admission Test (MCAT). To gain admission to an accredited college of medicine applicants must score competitively.

After graduating from four years of medical school, it is mandatory for a newly graduated physician to seek a residency or postgraduate specialty training program in a hospital. The graduate does this by applying for the National Resident Matching Program, a program developed in 1951 by representatives from the American Association of Medical Colleges (AAMC), the American Medical Association (AMA), and various hospital associations. This group acts as a national clearinghouse for matching the preferences of new graduates with the hospitals offering residencies.

The clearinghouse function gives a greater degree of freedom of choice for both the hospital and the medical student. Before the matching plan, graduating medical school students had to negotiate their own internships or residencies with individual hospitals. Since the students were notified by a specific date, it was often too late in the year to seek alternate internships if they were turned down. The matching plan allows for more students to be placed in approved residency programs (approved by the Council of Education of the AMA). Internships used to be the first year's postgraduate training for physicians. However, the internship category has now been eliminated in the AMA approved programs, and the first year is called the first year of residency. The matching plan has shown that an average of approximately 96 percent of the students are matched each year.[1] The results of the matching plan are announced in the early spring each year.

A hospital that has an approved residency program is more complex, and perhaps more interesting, than a hospital that does not offer educational programs. There are approximately 1,600 hospitals and other institutions in the country that have approved residences with over 81,000 residents in training. Also, there are 28 different specialty residency programs available and 39 subspecialties. The teaching hospital is essentially a living classroom. In these teaching hospitals the residents are referred to by their years of training. For example, a first-year resident is called a Post Graduate Year 1 or PGY1. Therefore, a PGY1 would be a low person on the resident (house staff) totempole; he/she is under the guidance of a senior resident who in turn is under the guidance of the chief resident in a given specialty. The chief residents in each specialty have the supervisory, managerial, and teaching responsibilities in the program. Generally, these residents are not licensed physicians, though in many states special temporary licenses are granted to practice within the institution that has the approved residency program. These residents are not independent contractors but are considered hospital employees. There was a time when the residents worked for a meager stipend. Now the residents receive respectable salaries for their efforts. The residents learn a great deal at the hospital, but they also give the hospital considerable in return by providing patient services.

After physicians complete their hospital residency programs, many seek to become certified in their specialties. This may require further training. Certification, referred to as Board of Certification, is under the jurisdiction of special boards such as the American Board of Surgery.

The objective of specialty boards and associations is to upgrade the qualifications of specialists. These boards and associations have increased the length of time needed for training, developed subspecialties, and sponsored numerous continuing education programs and professional journals. After rigorous examinations and proven abilities and practice, certification by a specialty board is indeed a recognition of professional competency. Fellowship in a specialty college is also a meaningful peer recognition of competence.

There has been a movement toward recertification by specialty boards in an attempt to ensure that physicians maintain an acceptable level of qualifications in their specialties. For instance, certification by the American Board of Surgery is valid for ten years. Physicians may apply for recertification as long as they are active, hold privileges in a hospital accredited by JCAHO, and have received satisfactory evaluations by the medical director. Those who pass the examination given by the American Board of Surgery are recertified.

CONTINUING MEDICAL EDUCATION

Following appointment to the medical staff of the hospital, the physician is obligated to provide proof of participation in a program of continuing medical education (CME). In fact, JCAHO standards stipulate that "the medical staff shall participate in a program of continuing education."[3] The scope and complexity of a physician's individual continuing education program or the hospital's program are left to each institution. It will vary depending on the resources at hand and the needs of the hospital. However, a hospital program must be relevant to the type of patient care delivered at the hospital. When a hospital does participate in a program, each staff member's participation should be documented and placed in that member's medical staff file.

ORGANIZED MEDICINE

In 1847, some 250 physicians, representing more than 40 medical societies and 28 colleges from 22 states, came together and founded the American Medical Association (AMA).[4] Pressure to begin the AMA stemmed from the poor quality of medical education in the United States at that time, the very brisk traffic in patent medicines and secret remedies, and the questionable ethics of many physicians of the time. The men who founded the AMA believed that a national association of physicians was needed to lead the crusade for improved medical education and patient care. The founding objectives of the AMA were two-fold: (1) to "promote the science and art of medicine and the betterment of public health," and (2) to promote "better health for all people and service to the professional needs of its membership."[5]

Membership in the AMA is open to any physician who has good standing in the local medical society. The AMA is a federation of some 54 constituent medical associations. These associations are in turn composed of more than 1,900 medical societies. Perhaps one of the AMA's greatest contributions to medicine is its "systematic and continuing gathering of data on new products, new findings, and new methods. This information is correlated, evaluated, summarized, and channeled to the AMA members."[6]

The AMA is involved in the legislative process and has become part of a strong hospital and medical lobby. In order to effectively respond to the regulatory and legal environment, the AMA has enhanced its original mission to include formulating national health care policies.

MEDICAL STAFF ORGANIZATION

The internal organization of the medical staff varies from hospital to hospital. Complex university or teaching hospitals differ from the smaller community hospitals. Because of the efforts of the JCAHO and its accreditation standards the differences are less today than in the past. The standards stipulate that there is to be a single organized medical staff that has overall responsibility for the quality of the professional services provided by individuals with clinical privileges, as well as the responsibility of accountability therefore to the governing body.[7]

Appointment to the medical staff is a formal process that is outlined in each hospital's medical staff bylaws, again with encouragement for standardization from the JCAHO. A brief outline of the appointment process that a doctor must go through follows:

- The applying physician completes a written application. The completed application is usually forwarded to the hospital CEO.
- The application is reviewed for completeness and verification and then sent for screening to the head of the specific department or specialty (e.g. medicine or surgery) to which the applicant is applying.
- The application is then forwarded to the medical staff's credentials committee, which reviews the physician's qualifications and past professional performance. It is at this point that the credentials committee may request a meeting with the applicant.
- Next the executive committee for the medical staff reviews and discusses the application. It sends its recommendation on to the hospital governing body.
- The board of trustees as a whole or through one of its committees reviews the application. The board will either accept, reject, or defer the application. If the application is questionable, requires more information, or needs discussion, it may be referred to the joint conference committee.
- The physician is usually notified by the CEO that the appointment has been approved or rejected. Any limitations on privileges requested may also be noted in the notice letter sent to the physician. In receiving approval a physician is granted certain clinical privileges (procedures the doctor is permitted to perform within the hospital). This is referred to as the individual's privilege delineation. The privilege delineation process is based on verifiable information made available to the credentials committee. A physician's demonstrated current competence in his/her discipline is the crucial determination of privileges. The privileges are listed on a form or placed on a record of some nature and kept on file in key places within the hospital—for example, within the operating room and the medical staff office.

The physician who has applied and has been admitted to the staff is appointed in two separate categories of membership: (1) to a clinical department or section and (2) with a status based on the extent of the physician's participation and privileges referred to as category. Staff membership status may be categorized as illustrated in Exhibit 9-1.

The organization of the hospital medical staff is divided into medical specialty departments and sections. For example, there may be departments of medicine, surgery, obstetrics and gynecology, and pediatrics. In larger hospitals these departments may be further subdivided into sections. Each clinical department has a physician designated as chief or director who is the medical administrative head. This person is generally selected through a process outlined in the medical staff

Exhibit 9-1 Categories of Medical Staff Membership

Attending Staff: Active staff members with full rights and privileges, voting prerogatives, and obligations to attend meetings, serve on committees, and handle emergency service responsibilities

Associate Staff: Staff members who have incomplete staff privileges and are in the transition from provisional active status

Provisional Staff: Staff members who were recently appointed and who have fewer privileges and responsibilities such as the inability to vote

Courtesy Staff: Staff members who do not frequently admit patients and who do not have the full obligations of active staff membership

Consulting Staff: Staff members with areas of specialization who consult with other staff members and who do not have the privileges of treating and admitting patients

Temporary Staff: Staff members who are only given privileges for a designated period of time

Source: Reprinted from *Health Care Administration: Principles and Practices* by Lawrence F. Wolper and Jesus J. Pena, p. 297, Aspen Publishers, Inc, © 1987.

bylaws. Usually this is done either through election by departmental members or by appointment by the hospital board of trustees.

CLOSED AND OPEN MEDICAL STAFFS

Historically, individual hospitals have controlled their own admissions to medical staff. However, in recent years hospitals' autonomy has eroded in this area. A closed medical staff is one that closely monitors and restricts any new applicants to the staff or to a department of the staff. This is generally done with the concurrence of the hospital board of trustees. When a hospital does permit a closed medical staff, it is usually based upon considerations related to the quality of and need for patient care within the hospital and within the community. There may also be closed medical staffs within selected departments or sections in the hospital—the two most notable examples are the radiology and pathology departments. In these hospital-based departments, the hospital signs an agreement with a physician or a professional group to allow exclusive services in the department. The courts have generally found this to be a legal arrangement if such agreements are based upon significant medical and administrative considerations. Closed medical staff issues are frequently addressed in the courts under the Federal Anti-Trust Laws. Additionally, since the Federal Trade Commission (FTC) has the power to promulgate rules and regulations defining unfair practices in this area, it is reasonable to assume that it will be a predominant enforcement agency relative to medical staff admissions in years to come. An open staff essentially admits all qualified physicians who meet the hospital's guidelines.

MEDICAL STAFF COMMITTEES

The JCAHO standards dictate that "the medical staff shall develop and adopt bylaws, rules, and regulations to establish a framework of self-government and a means for accountability to the governing body."[8] The bylaws outline the form of self-government of the medical staff. The medical staff conducts its business through committees. The committee chairpersons are either selected by members of the staff or appointed by the president of the staff.

One of the most important committees is the medical staff executive committee. It continues the medical staff business in the interim between general staff meetings. Generally, the executive committee is composed of the officers of the staff and a number of elected members from the staff. Typically, this committee meets monthly conducting the business of the medical staff. The hospital CEO usually attends. The medical executive committee coordinates various committees, and rules that effect the different clinical departments of the staff. The credentials committee, the medical records committee, the tissue committee, and the medical audit and quality committee are other key committees of the staff. The credentials committee has the responsibility to review the qualifications of new physicians applying for membership. This committee also reviews the credentials of medical staff members who must be reappointed. Reappointment is usually either once a year or every other year. The credentials committee could also be the committee to investigate breaches of ethics or misconduct among the members of the medical staff. This committee reports directly to the executive committee.

Since medical records have become the principal instrument for review of quality assurance in hospitals, the medical committee has taken on a more important function in recent years. Initially the medical records committee was responsible for reviewing the forms that were used in the medical records. It now also reviews the quantity and quality of patient records as written by physicians, nurses, or other associated health professionals in the hospital. It also serves as a monitor of the physicians who may have delinquent medical records. This committee works closely with the hospital's medical records administrator.

An efficient medical audit committee and a well-functioning tissue committee traditionally have been key instruments in assessing quality. The tissue committee provides a vehicle to confirm the diagnosis for surgical cases and acts as a control on unnecessary surgery. Practicing surgeons plus a member of the hospital pathology department make up the membership. The tissue committee reviews all surgical cases to determine, based on the review of tissue taken from the patient, whether the surgery was necessary. Tissue removed from an operation is forwarded to the pathology laboratory for postoperative diagnosis and review.

The medical audit committee, sometimes called the quality assurance committee, safeguards quality in the hospital. This committee is generally made up of physicians with some staff administrative support. It reviews the practice of medicine in all disciplines. Attention is given to clinical outcomes and problem solving.

THE MEDICAL DIRECTOR

Hospitals usually employ full-time medical directors. Management apparently feels this is the most appropriate way to fulfill its responsibility for quality care in the institution. Not surprisingly, some medical staffs see this trend as a threat to their self-governance and as an administrative encroachment into medical staff affairs. Generally the medical director is a top-level management employee whose position may be full-time or part-time. If part-time, the medical director may also see patients and therefore could be a member of the medical staff. The medical director's role is to evaluate clinical performance and to enforce hospital policy related to quality care. However, as in other management jobs, the role may be expanded to include other activities.

ALLIED HEALTH PERSONNEL

There continues to be an increasing number of nonphysicians and nondentists applying for clinical privileges within the hospital, including but not limited to podiatrists, chiropractors, physician assistants, nurse practitioners, nurse midwives, and psychologists. By applying for medical staff privileges, some of these groups have raised the question of how they fit into the hospital medical staff.

Historically, with the backing of laws and regulations, hospitals have excluded these groups from practicing within the hospital. Generally, state regulations regarding nurse practitioners and physician assistants indicate that a physician must supervise their work. The American Medical Association basically agrees with the American Hospital Association on this issue and feels that full medical staff privileges should be restricted to physicians and dentists. The Joint Commission on Accreditation of Hospital Organizations has been somewhat more liberal with regard to podiatrists and has delineated what it believes a podiatrist can do within a hospital. The JCAHO permits other duly licensed health care professionals to practice in hospitals under the supervision of a practitioner who has clinical privileges. The case law on the privilege question is not absolutely clear, and it is reasonable to assume that each individual issue may be decided based upon state statutes and license practice laws within each state.

Table 9-1 Legal Restrictions on Physicians

Area of Law	Prohibitions
Federal Antitrust Statutes	Prohibits collaboration between unrelated parties to engage in price fixing or restraint of trade
State Corporate Practice of Medicine Laws	Prohibits ownership or management of clinical aspects of physician practice by persons or organizations other than physicians
IRS Code for Not-for-Profit Organizations	Prohibits payments to individuals having a personal and private interest in a tax-exempt organization
Medicare/Medicaid Fraud and Abuse	Prohibits payment or receipt of remuneration of any kind for the referral of Medicare and Medicaid patients
State Fee-Splitting Laws	Prohibits rebates or kickbacks to physicians in return for referrals

Source: Adapted from *Physician Bonding, Volume 1: Overview Strategies Coast to Coast* by Health Care Advisory Board, p. 9, 1987.

LEGAL RESTRICTIONS ON PHYSICIANS

Today physicians are legally and professionally restricted in their practice of medicine and in their commercial ventures. Table 9-1 highlights some paramount legal concerns for physicians.

Physicians' professional conduct is monitored closely, too. The Health Care Quality Improvement Act of 1986 set up a National Practitioner Data Bank in 1990 to prevent physicians, as well as other healthcare professionals, from hiding acts of malpractice and professional misbehavior by moving to other states. Sources of data include hospitals, malpractice insurers, and state licensing boards. Hospitals must check the data bank during their credentialing process.

NOTES

1. Robert M. Farrier, "National Intern Resident Matching Program," *Hospital Progress,* November 1973, p. 12.

2A. *1990-1991 Directory of Graduate Medical Education Programs* (Chicago, Ill.: American Hospital Association, 1990).

2B. *Socio-Economic Factbook for Surgery* (Chicago, Ill.: American College of Surgeons, 1989), p. 9.

3. Schulz and Johnson, *Management of Hospitals,* p. 74.

4. Leslie J. DeGroot, *Medical Care: Social and Organizationing Aspects* (Springfield, Ill.: Charles C. Thomas, 1966), p. 438.

5. Ibid, p. 438.

6. Ibid, p. 442.

7. American Hospital Association, *Hospital Week* (Chicago, Ill.: December 1978), Vol. 14, No. 49.

8. Joint Commission on Accreditation of Hospitals, *Accreditation Manual for Hospitals—1980 Edition* (Chicago, Ill.: 1979), p. 93.

Nursing Services

Chapter 10

Key Terms

Mother of modern nursing • Nursing schools • American Nursing Association (AMA) • National League for Nursing (NLN) • Director of nurses (DON) • Vice president of nursing • Nursing supervisor • Nursing unit • Head nurse • Staff nurses • Auxiliary nursing personnel • Nurses' station • Nursing shifts • Intensive care unit (ICU) • Coronary care unit (CCU) • Nursing standards • Case nursing • Functional nursing • Team nursing • Primary care nursing • Acuity system • Scheduling • Staffing • Telemonitoring • Bedside terminal

---

INTRODUCTION

Hospitalized patients should receive quality, courteous, and considerate care given by skillful, understanding personnel. The primary department to meet this goal is the nursing service department. Nurses account for the single largest health professional group in the country. In 1988, there were 2,033,000 professional nurses of whom 1,627,000 were employed in nursing.[1] Of this, a large number are employed in hospitals. At the same time, there were approximately 585,600 doctors.[2] The nursing service department accounts for approximately 25 percent of all hospital operating expenses and can represent upward to 35 to 40 percent of total hospital salary expenses.

EARLY TRADITIONS

The early history of nursing was influenced by both individuals (e.g., Florence Nightingale) and institutions such as the Roman Catholic Church and the military.

75

Perhaps the best known person associated with the history of nursing is Florence Nightingale, whose work during the Crimean War gave nursing a more respectable image. She became known as the "mother of modern nursing." After the war, Florence Nightingale founded the Florence Nightingale Nursing School in connection with St. Thomas Hospital in London in 1859.

Schools for training American nurses can be found as far back as 1798. However, American schools that embodied the principles of Florence Nightingale's school in London were established much later. The first such school was the New England Hospital for Women and Children founded in Boston in 1872. This was followed in 1873 by the Bellevue Hospital School of Nursing in New York City. The Massachusetts General Hospital in Boston opened its school of nursing in 1873, also. Over the next 50 years, there were some 2,000 nursing schools established in the United States. Today, there are 1,429 nursing schools in the United States.[3] These schools' programs include diploma programs based in hospitals, two-year associate degree programs in community colleges, and four-year baccalaureate programs in colleges and universities.

NURSING EDUCATION

Changes in the well-established Nightingale nursing education model emerged following World War II. With the acute shortage of professional registered nurses (RNs), the licensed practical or vocational nurse (LPN or LVN) came into vogue. The number of nurses' aides also continued to rise. Meanwhile, educational programs for the registered nurses began to change, especially in the 1960s. During this time, the three-year, hospital-diploma, nursing education programs began to be phased out because of the high cost of nursing education and pressures from the American Nurses Association for a baccalaureate or associate degree education.

Nurses now have a variety of education/experience combinations from which to select (see Table 10-1). Registered nurses can earn a Ph.D., which usually takes more than seven years of academic work interspersed with practical experience. Nurses with advanced degrees may work as clinical nurse specialists, nurse clinicians, nurse practitioners, nurse midwives, or nurse anesthetists. On the other hand, a prospective nurse may choose a one-year academic program integrated with practical experience. These nurses are called licensed practical or vocational nurses (LPNs or LVNs).

All professional and practical nurses must be licensed by the state in which they practice nursing. Every state determines its own eligibility criteria for licensing and relicensing and also is responsible for suspending and revoking licenses. Usually completed educational requirements and the passing of the state's board examination are necessary for initial licensing although only payment of a small fee is required for relicensing if it is done before the original license expires.

Table 10-1 Educational Requirements for Nurses

Educational Level	Training Required Beyond High School	Curriculum	Training Site
Registered nurse— Ph.D. and D.N.S., (Doctor of Nursing Science)	3 to 5 years post-baccalaureate	Academic program integrated with practical work throughout the years	University
Registered nurse— master's degree	5 to 6 academic years	1- to 2-year academic program integrated with practical work	University, hospital, and community health agencies
Registered nurse— baccalaureate degree	4 years and summer sessions	4-year academic program integrated with practical experience	University, hospital, and community health agencies
Registered nurse— diploma	27–36 months	1-year academic work, 2 years of practical experience with clinical courses	Hospital
Registered nurse— associate degree	2 years	2-year academic program integrated with practical experience	Junior college
Licensed practical or vocational nurse (LPN or LVN)	1 year	1-year academic program integrated with practical experience	Vocational technical school and hospital

There are two large and influential national professional nursing association groups. The American Nurses Association (ANA) founded in 1896 is a federation of 54 constituent associations, including those in the 50 states, the District of Columbia, and Puerto Rico. As a group, they promote legislation and speak out for nurses on legislative action programs. The other influential nursing association is the National League for Nursing (NLN) founded in 1951. This is a community-centered group that brings together people in the health and welfare fields with the lay community to work primarily for the improvement of nursing service and nursing education. The NLN's membership is composed of registered nurses, practical nurses, nurses' aides, doctors, and hospital administrators—all of whom have a professional interest in nursing.

DEPARTMENT ORGANIZATION

Approximately 40 percent of all hospital employees work in the nursing service department. Each of the many varied positions in the department has a job description. In each hospital, the department must have specific job descriptions and procedure manuals.

The nursing service department is organized in a pyramid fashion very much like the hospital as a whole. The primary responsibility rests with the director of the nursing service department, referred to as the director of nurses (DON) or vice president of nursing. Directors are usually selected because of their management abilities; they are often registered nurses with advanced degrees (sometimes in the specific discipline of nursing service administration). Often, the director has one or two assistant directors to aid in the management of the department. The title of supervisor is frequently given to the position held by a registered nurse who supervises or directs the activities of two or more nursing units. The supervisor may manage and direct the many nursing service activities during the evenings, nights, or weekends; thus, the titles of night supervisor, weekend supervisor, or day supervisor are often applied. If a hospital has a nursing school, the director of nursing is often responsible for both the nursing service and the nursing school. Or the nursing school may have its own director who reports to the director of nurses. If there is no school of nursing, the training function of the nursing department is usually assigned to an assistant director who is responsible for the education, orientation, and continuing inservice education of all employees in the department of nursing.

The nursing service department is also organized along geographical lines. Each of the nursing service responsibilities for patient care is decentralized to a specific location in the hospital called a nursing unit or patient care unit. Certain responsibilities and functions to operate a nursing unit are assigned to a head nurse. A head nurse supervises the personnel in a patient care unit. A head nurse may also be referred to by other titles, such as nurse manager or patient care manager. This person is accountable for the quality of the nursing care on the unit, controls the supplies, and schedules the staff. Usually the head nurse has a series of staff nurses. The staff nurses are assigned specific responsibilities for the nursing care of patients on the nursing unit.

A large number of employees in the nursing service are grouped under the title of auxiliary nursing personnel; these include nurses' aides, orderlies, and technicians. Auxiliary nursing personnel generally go through at least a hospital orientation training program before assuming their nursing duties with patients. Some states require a formal training program for nurses' aides. They do not need to be graduates of a formal education program, nor are they licensed or certified. These personnel generally are assigned duties by the graduate nurse, staff nurse, or head nurse.

Many of the individual nursing units have a host of clerical functions to be performed. Unit clerks assigned to nursing service handle the enormous quantity of paperwork, answer telephones, direct visitors, help with hospital requisitions for patients and supplies, and perform other similar duties. These clerks usually work directly under the supervision of a head nurse.

THE NURSING UNIT

As noted earlier, the nursing care of the hospital is organized in a decentralized fashion into patient care units or nursing units. The size of nursing units vary. They can be very small, with 8- to 10-bed units for specialized care, or they can be large, with 60- to 70-bed units. Perhaps the most common size is between 20 and 40 beds per unit.[4] Nursing units generally operate on three shifts to cover the 24-hour period. They usually operate as a day shift between 7:00 A.M. and 3:00 P.M. The evening shift, called the evening tour, runs from 3:00 P.M. to 11:00 P.M., and the night shift runs from 11:00 P.M. to 7:00 A.M. Some units operate on two 12-hour shifts—7 A.M. to 7 P.M. and from 7 P.M. to 7 A.M. There are disagreements over the most effective way to organize the distribution of patient rooms on a nursing unit. Most rooms are semiprivate and accommodate two patients. There are also private or single-bed accommodation rooms. Usually there is at least one single-bed accommodation room on a nursing unit that is designed and reserved for patients with illnesses warranting isolation.

The size of the nursing unit and the distribution of single and multibed rooms are considered before a unit is built. Consideration is given to the cost of construction of the unit, the duplication of equipment, and how much nursing service time will be required to staff the unit. If the unit is spacious and rooms are distributed at a distance from the central nursing point, the staff must continually travel to reach a patient and supplies. Although the unit may look pleasing, it may not be work

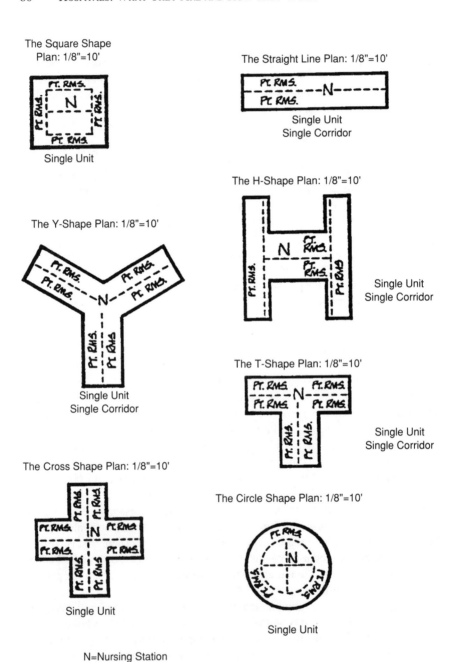

The Square Shape
Plan: 1/8"=10'

Single Unit

The Straight Line Plan: 1/8"=10'

Single Unit
Single Corridor

The Y-Shape Plan: 1/8"=10'

Single Unit
Single Corridor

The H-Shape Plan: 1/8"=10'

Single Unit
Single Corridor

The T-Shape Plan: 1/8"=10'

Single Unit
Single Corridor

The Cross Shape Plan: 1/8"=10'

Single Unit

The Circle Shape Plan: 1/8"=10'

Single Unit

N=Nursing Station

Figure 10-1 Various Shapes of Floor Plans with Alternative Designs

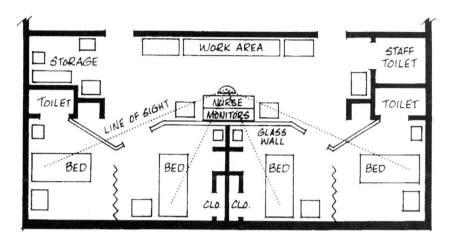

Figure 10-2 Nursing Station Floor Plan in Rectangular Configuration

---

efficient. There are a variety of designs and configurations for nursing units. Some of the more common nursing unit layouts are shown in Figure 10-1. Figures 10-2 and 10-3 show the typical layouts for critical care units. Whether a rectangular or circular configuration is used, it is imperative that patients can be seen from the nursing station. Usually the patient rooms are cubicles with curtains or rooms with glass walls.

Where the patient rooms are private or semiprivate, they will vary in size. It has been suggested that the minimum size for a private room should be not less than 125 square feet with a minimum width of at least 12 feet, 6 inches.[5] As to the two-bed accommodation, a minimum of 160 square feet is usually provided with the beds separated by cubicle curtains. For a four-bed room, the minimum is generally considered to be 320 square feet. The hospital bed is generally 86 inches long, 36 inches wide, about 27 inches from the floor, and can be varied electrically or mechanically into different positions.

OTHER COMPONENTS OF THE NURSING UNIT

Among the elements found on nursing units is the nurses' station, which tends to be the focal point of administrative activity. The nurses' station is generally where the nurses keep their records and is centrally located to all the activities of the entire nursing unit. On a nursing unit there is also a medicine preparation room area. Every nursing unit has a utility room. This is a work space where clean supplies, instruments, and equipment and "used" or "dirty" equipment that has been used by the patients are stored. Usually there is also a small pantry, or sometimes

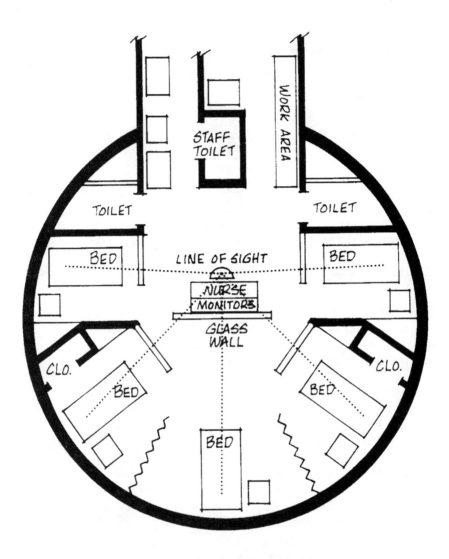

Figure 10-3 Nursing Station Floor Plan in Circular Configuration

even a large kitchen, on the nursing unit, depending on the method used by the hospital to deliver its dietary services. If the food is prepackaged or preplated before coming to the nursing unit, a smaller pantry will suffice. If the food is delivered to the nursing unit in bulk fashion and distributed, a larger kitchen may be necessary. There is also a nurses' lounge where nurses take breaks, eat meals, receive inservices, and give change of shift reports. Other rooms that might be found on nursing units are a common toilet/bath area (if they are not available individually in the patient rooms), a consultation room where physicians and the families of the patients may meet, and treatment rooms. Some units may also have a pleasant place for visitors to sit down with the patients outside of their rooms.

SPECIAL CARE UNITS

Special care units have developed with today's increased technology and modern medical advances. Over the last decade, special care units have multiplied and matured. The sophisticated modern hospital may have a variety of special care facilities to manage and to maintain patients with special illnesses and injuries. These facilities may include intensive care units for medicine and surgery, special cardiac care units, hemodialysis or renal dialysis centers, inpatient psychiatric units, inpatient alcoholic and drug addiction units, pediatric units, and skilled nursing facilities for long-term care. A special unit need not be based in the hospital; it may be constituted as a hospital home care program.

Intensive Care Units

The most common type of special care unit in the hospital is the general medical/surgical intensive care unit (ICU). There are over 4,200 such units in the hospital systems of this country.[6] The ICU units were established to meet clinical demands of the hospitalized patients and their physicians. Their purpose is to manage the critically ill patient who is in a precarious clinical status and requires "eagle eye" supervision. The ICUs handle both surgical and medical cases. ICU cases could be patients in shock, stroke victims, or persons with heart failures, serious infections, respiratory distress, and so forth. The establishment of separate ICU units in hospitals was a major step forward in modern hospital care. By marshalling the hospital's resources in one geographic area, it is much easier to provide efficient high quality care. Not only are sophisticated equipment and instrumentation available in ICUs, but a highly concentrated nursing staff is also used. These nursing personnel may have successfully completed critical care training at the hospital and have had medical and surgical nursing care work experience.

A special offshoot of the ICU is the neonatal intensive care unit that specializes in the management of critical health problems in the newborn. Caring for the critically ill newborn requires a specially trained nurse and physician. The neonatal intensive care units have had great success in the handling of premature infants, giving them a new lease on life.

Coronary Care Units

The ICUs in hospitals gave birth to coronary care units (CCUs). The CCUs may be quite familiar to the ordinary health care consumer since they have grown in popularity over the past ten years. Today, nearly all of the medical-surgical hospitals in the United States have some CCU capacities, if one includes those facilities that have CCU capacities in their ICUs. There are over 1,100 discrete and specialized CCUs in operation today.[7]

The CCUs do for cardiac patients what the ICUs do for severe medical and surgical patients. However, the CCU has not had such a dramatic impact on saving lives as has the ICU, however, cardiac disease is growing and the need for hospitals to treat the patients has placed CCU units on the "front line."

For both ICUs and CCUs, it is usual to have a medical director assigned either full-time, part-time, or rotating to medically manage the units. Individual attending physicians manage their own patients. However, because there is a medical director, the attending physicians have to relinquish some of the old concept of total and complete control over their patients and realize that their care is a shared responsibility in these two intensive care units.

The nurse's role in these units is critical. The nurses should be intelligent observers, and they must be able to interpret changes in a patient. Under critical circumstances, they might have to diagnose and even treat the patient. One of the prime objectives of the CCU is to detect early signs of impending cardiac distress so that it can be treated before cardiac arrest takes place.

Nonacute Special Care Units

There are a variety of special care units that are not geared for life-threatening situations. One of the best examples is the renal dialysis centers that have been increasing in number over the last decade. The renal dialysis centers provide artificial kidney support for patients whose kidneys have stopped functioning properly. These units, unlike the CCUs and ICUs, provide long-term care needs for patients. Other nonacute special care units include psychiatric units and inpatient alcohol and drug-related units.

Long-Term Care Facilities

Given the aging population and the number of patients who need nursing home care after hospitalization, many hospitals have become involved in long-term care programs. More and more hospitals have long-term or nursing home beds or hospital-based nursing facilities within their institutions.

Today, 990 hospitals have long-term care skilled nursing units in their institutions.[9] The patients in these facilities are generally recovering from strokes, severe orthopedic accidents, or severe medical illnesses. There are two generally recognized kinds of nursing homes or kinds of care (1) skilled nursing facilities (SNFs), and (2) lower-level nursing facilities called intermediate care facilities (ICFs).

MODES OF NURSING CARE DELIVERY

Today there are four commonly used modes of nursing delivery: case method of nursing, functional nursing, team nursing, and primary care nursing.

Case Nursing

The case method of nursing is one of the earliest forms of nursing care. In this system, the nurse individually plans and administers the care of a patient. This is done on a one-to-one basis. The case method has persisted over the years in a couple of nursing areas. It is used today as the model of nursing in nursing schools because it allows nursing students to be taught the "idealized" patient care system. It is also used in acute care settings, such as intensive care, and may be used on the general nursing unit in private-duty nursing situations.

Functional Nursing

Starting in the 1920s and continuing into the 1940s, nurses became aware of the studies and developments in the functional division of labor in industry, as seen in the assembly line approach to manufacturing used by Henry Ford and other industrialists. Nurses then applied these time and motion studies to their own discipline. Essentially, functional nursing uses a pyramid organization to look at the division of labor. Under such an arrangement, each of the members of the nursing staff on the unit has technical aspects of that member's job identified; with this knowledge, each unit member is given specific functions or tasks to perform on the unit. For example, one nurse might administer medications, another would give all the treatments, a third might take all the temperatures and blood pressures of patients, and a fourth might prepare those patients going to surgery or x-ray. All would give baths, make beds, and try to meet the patient's psychological and emotional needs. The simpler tasks would be given to the less trained nursing personnel and the more complex tasks, to the registered nurses. Functional nursing is often utilized on the evening and night shifts where the number of tasks has generally been reduced.

Team Nursing

Team nursing began around World War II when there was a shortage of registered nurses (RNs). In the absence of RNs, hospitals had to use technicians, vocational nurses, and nurses' aides. Frequently, the less trained nursing personnel were put under the supervision of a more highly trained registered nurse, who was called the team leader. This team was asked to provide care to a group of patients on the nursing unit. Ideally, the team leader was the best prepared person and was expected to facilitate the team in formulating and carrying out the nursing care plans for every patient assigned to the team. Team nursing fits very well into the pyramid structure of the hospital organization.

Primary Care Nursing

Primary care nursing has some of the characteristics of the case method of nursing, in that one registered nurse is assigned to each patient. However, unlike the case method of nursing, the nurse assigned to the patient is not responsible only for one shift of work. The primary care nurse is responsible for the care of the patient for 24 hours a day, seven days a week. It is the primary care nurse's responsibility to assess a patient's nursing needs. The primary care nurse collaborates with other health professionals, including the physician, and formulates a plan of nursing care for which the nurse becomes responsible and accountable. The primary care nurse provides all of the patient's custodial care needs such as bathing and feeding as well as the patient's skilled care needs such as the administration of medications. The primary care nurse may delegate certain responsibilities for executing that plan on the other shifts, but the delegation is accomplished by means of other nursing care plans, including written notes and recordings. Carrying out the plan is never done through a supervisor or third party; thus an important element of primary care nursing is the "triple A nurse." The triple A nurse is *au*tonomous, has the *a*uthority, and is held *a*ccountable for the nursing care of the patient.

TERMS AND STANDARDS

An understanding of precisely which nursing standard was used when the nursing department's budget and staffing schedule were established is an important element in nursing service. A nursing standard or nursing norm is defined as the amount of time and resources needed or considered desirable for each patient in a 24-hour period in order to give the type of care judged appropriate. The American Hospital Association and the National League for Nursing identified various nursing standards as early as 1950. Nursing managers should be able to ask such questions as: Is the ratio of registered nurses to other personnel in the department too high? Are there too many or too few licensed practical nurses for the situation? Is there another way to assign duties in order to improve budgetary performance?

Financial managers should know that when nursing service expenses are low or below budget, a detailed look at the nursing staff patterns may be required. Perhaps student nurses have been utilized in place of staff nurses. Perhaps private duty nurses were attached to some other cost center and were used in place of regular staff nurses. Perhaps inadequate information was available at the time the budget was established. Perhaps the department was unable to fill all budgeted positions. Perhaps the onduty nursing staff is carrying an unfair load. To analyze all these specific circumstances, a financial manager must have an understanding of certain nursing definitions and terms that are widely accepted in the nursing service area.

The patient, upon entering the hospital, in effect agrees to an unwritten contract that the care the hospital renders will be adequate. The questions are: What is adequate care? How many registered nurses and ancillary nursing staff are required to provide adequate care? These are important questions that are central to the nursing department's mission. They should be answered and evaluated only in the light of a nursing standard.

STAFFING

Nurse staffing is the result of determining the appropriate number of full-time equivalent nursing personnel (FTEs) by each nursing skill class (RNs, LPNs, nurses' aides) to properly operate each nursing unit. Given the great contrast in the levels of nursing care required by different patients, and the large manpower needs of a nursing unit, staffing is a real challenge for a nursing department. The key to determining how much staff and what proper qualifications are needed is using patient acuity systems.

Patient acuity systems classify patients into care categories and quantify the nursing effort required. Patients' physical, technical, psychological, social, and teaching requirements are assessed in determining acuity levels. A common type of classification system is a list of critical indicators or condition indicators such as sensory deficit, oxygen therapy, and wound care, that are separately rated and then summed up to determine the patient's care category. Care categories include routine care, moderate care, complete care, and continuous care. For each patient care category the total nursing care time is quantified by the nursing department.

Many patient acuity systems are computerized. Daily, weekly, and seasonal variations must be considered in staffing arrangement. Hospitals may use "float nurses," part-time nursing pool personnel, and agency contracted nurses (rent-a-nurse) in addition to the hospital's full-time nursing staff to meet patient care needs.

SCHEDULING

Once the nursing department agrees on the standards to be used to staff the nursing unit, and the nursing administration agrees on the type of nursing (nursing modalities) best suited for the hospital, the challenge to nursing then is to schedule nursing personnel so that the patients receive the necessary care at the time they require it. Nurse scheduling is defined as determining when each member of the nursing staff will be on duty and on which shift each will work. Scheduling should take into account weekends, length of an individual's work stretches, and nursing requests for vacation and time off. Scheduling is typically done for a period of four or six weeks, and the scheduling is frequently tailored to each individual nursing unit. There are three commonly used approaches to nurse scheduling: the traditional, the cyclical, and the computer-aided traditional approaches.

Traditional Scheduling

In traditional scheduling, the nurse schedulers start from scratch each period (week, month). Generally, the head nurse makes the scheduling decisions by taking pencil and paper in hand and looking at the roster of personnel who are available to work on specified dates and for certain durations. This places in the head nurse's hands a great deal of responsibility for the quality and quantity of coverage on the nursing unit. The major advantage of this traditional approach is its flexibility. Since nurses begin essentially from scratch each period, they are able to adjust to changes of environment on the nursing unit quite quickly. Some of traditional scheduling's disadvantages include spottiness in coverage at times and uneven quality of coverage. Unless policies in the nursing administration leave some flexibility in the process, uneven staffing could also lead to higher personnel cost.

Cyclical Scheduling

Cyclical scheduling is a system that covers a certain period of time, perhaps one or three months. This block of time is the cycle or scheduling period. Once having agreed on a definite period, the scheduling in the cycle simply repeats itself period after period. The advantage of cyclical scheduling is that it provides even coverage with a higher quality of coverage determined for each nursing unit. Special requests would interfere with the coverage, which could impact the quality of staffing. The major disadvantage to cyclical scheduling is that it is inflexible compared to the traditional system and is not able to adjust rapidly to changes in the nursing unit environment. The ability to adjust is important, since change characterizes so many nursing units. The environment in which cyclical scheduling seems to work best is one in which the number of patients and their needs are fairly constant and the nurses are stable and do not rotate between shifts. New nurses can be hired into any open cyclical slot with very little difficulty.

Computer-Aided Traditional Scheduling

The third approach to scheduling uses the computer to help the traditional method of scheduling. This permits mathematical programming to be applied to traditional nurse scheduling. This system provides the traditional approach with more flexibility, and it also reduces the operating costs involved in calculating and in working with the schedule. To some extent, the computer centralizes the scheduling process. If mathematical models are properly used, the computer can produce high-quality schedules. The system will also facilitate the incorporation of standard personnel policies into the schedule, and the policies can be applied uniformly over all nursing units. It will also add more stability to the entire nursing department. The advantages of computerized scheduling are most dramatically apparent in situations where nurses rotate frequently among shifts and where nursing environments are subject to chronic change. Computer-aided, centralized schedules minimize the time spent on preparing and maintaining schedules.

TELEMONITORING AND BEDSIDE TERMINALS

Along with burgeoning technological innovation and the use of patient acuity levels, telemonitoring equipment, bedside terminals, and automated clinical records are being used by nurses. Telemonitoring equipment may vary from hospital to hospital depending on the complexity of the unit, the needs of the patients, and the resources of the hospital. The equipment can be used for routine evaluation of blood pressure, pulse, respiration, temperature, and other selected physical and physiological conditions. In the intensive care unit, it is important to have built-in alarm systems that will warn the staff of critical changes in the patient's condition. Types of cardiac monitoring equipment include oscilloscopes at the patient's bedside, supplemented by heart rate meters with audio and visual alarms, pacemakers with automatic or manual controls, and electrocardiograph recordings. At the nurses' station, there is usually a central panel that includes oscilloscope and heart rate meters with audio and visual alarms.

Unlike telemonitory equipment, bedside terminals involve nursing interaction. Nurses directly enter and retrieve patients' clinical data using bedside computer terminals. Data may include vital signs, lab results, and medications given. By utilizing bedside terminals, nurses are more productive and have more time to devote to patients and other nursing functions. Also, by capturing data at the source or point of care, patient information is more accurate. It is ideal to integrate bedside terminals with the hospital's information system. This facilitates communication between nurses and other allied health professionals and results in more responsive patient care.

The outcome of bedside terminals is an automated clinical record. This is a substitute for the traditional patient chart. A patient's clinical data is part of an integrated system that allows easy access to nurses, physicians, and allied health professionals.

NURSE MANPOWER ISSUES

As a result of labor force changes, there are shortages of nurses as well as other allied health professionals in certain areas of the country. Since the hospital is a labor intensive industry, shortages can have a major impact on the operation of a hospital. Hospitals are meeting this challenging manpower issue through the implementation of creative strategies. Some of these strategies include giving bonuses, using clinical career ladders to motivate and reward nurses involved in direct patient care, allowing nurses to budget for their unit, broadening job responsibility and autonomy, providing inservices, and offering child day-care services.

NOTES

1. The U.S. Dept. of Health & Human Services, Health Resources Services Administration Division of Nurses provided the 1988 data.

2. *Physician Characteristics & Distribution in the U.S.* (Chicago, Ill.: American Medical Association, 1988)

3. Nursing Data Source, National League for Nursing (New York, N.Y.: 1990).

4. John McGiboney, *Principles of Hospital Administration* (New York, N.Y.: G.P. Putnam's Sons, 1969), p. 435.

5. Ibid, p. 436.

6. American Hospital Association, *Hospital Statistics* (Chicago, Ill.: AHA, 1990–91).

7. Ibid.

8. Ronald Gotz and Arthur Kaufman, *The People's Hospital Book* (New York, N.Y.: Crown Publishers, Inc., 1978), p. 168.

9. *AHA Hospital Statistics* (Chicago, Ill.: 1990), p. 222.

Part V

Tests and Results

Chapter 11

Key Ancillary Services

Key Terms

Ancillary • Surgical specimens • Pathologist • Registered medical technologist • Medical imaging • William Röentgen • Computerized tomography (CT) • Magnetic resonance imaging • Ultrasound • Nuclear medicine • Laboratory information systems • Radiologist • Freestanding imaging centers • Nurse anesthetist • Informed consent for surgery • Anesthesiologist

---

INTRODUCTION

The hospital's ancillary departments may also be called professional service departments. Literally, ancillary means a department that assists the physician in the diagnosis or treatment of the patient. Ancillary is defined as a cost (having expenses) and revenue center (able to bill the patient for services) within the hospital which requires, either by regulation or third-party urging, either that a physician direct the department or that a physician provide guidance and supervision over the department. In other words, what differentiates an ancillary service department from other hospital departments is that it is able to charge the patient directly, thereby generating revenue for the hospital, and it must be under the direction of a physician.

Ancillary departments are very complex because their charge structure is different and consists of many individual tests. In addition, the departments have highly sophisticated equipment and a variety of well-trained technical staff. Another factor that makes these departments complex for management is physician compensation. There are a variety of ways in which the physicians who direct these departments may be reimbursed.

A typical large community hospital will have the following ancillary departments: clinical laboratory, radiology (x-ray or medical imaging), physical therapy, inhalation therapy, anesthesiology, EKG (electrocardiography, heart station), and EEG (electroencephalography). To illustrate the function of the organization and how ancillary departments relate to the physicians and to the patients, the following sections provide some details and an analysis of three major ancillary departments: clinical laboratories, radiology, and anesthesiology.

CLINICAL LABORATORIES DEPARTMENT

Clinical laboratories, another term for pathology departments, are of rather recent origin. Yet, in their relatively short period of existence, they have undergone tremendous growth. Just before World War I, a typical hospital pathology department was small and ill-equipped. Pathologists spent most of their time doing simple urinalyses, blood counts, and a few chemical determinations in bacteriology. Only a few surgical specimens (tissue removed by the physician during surgery) were examined, and only a few autopsies were performed. After World War I, the pathology and clinical laboratory departments began to grow. Physicians, having learned the value of pathology services from their war experiences, began to demand such services in civilian hospitals.

Between 1875 and 1900, bacteriology reached its golden age. In fact, most of the important pathogenic microorganisms were isolated in this period. However, it was several years before these techniques became widely applied. It was not until 1937 that blood banking was used as a practical procedure in hospitals. Following World War II, additional growth occurred. New knowledge on how to expose health and disease problems proliferated. Diagnostic radioisotopes, exfoliative cytology, molecular diseases, practical virology, and fluorescent studies were introduced.

Functions

A hospital's clinical laboratory has a number of functions, but its primary purpose is to provide information to assist physicians and other members of the health team in the diagnosis, prevention, and treatment of disease. This primary mission is accomplished by performing tests in the laboratory. Fields in which laboratory tests are performed include bacteriology, biochemistry, histology, serology, and cytology.

The clinical laboratory is responsible for the blood bank as well. Blood banking as a regular service in hospitals is concerned with such blood procedures as crossmatching, compatibility testing, and the preparation and storage of blood prior to transfusion. Another major concern for the blood bank is screening for contaminated blood products. An additional responsibility for the clinical laboratory is the operation of the hospital's morgue. Other related functions of the clinical laboratory depend on the size and complexity of the hospital; these can involve training programs and research.

One of the important ways a laboratory improves the quality of medicine is through its formal reports, especially on post-mortem examinations and on examinations of tissues removed in surgical operations (surgical specimens). Tissue committees serve as a classic quality control mechanism whereby practicing surgeons can measure and improve their clinical performance in the hospital.

Organization

The department is organized under the leadership and directorship of a pathologist. This is a licensed physician who specializes in the practice of pathology and is usually eligible for certification or certified by the American Board of Pathology in either clinical or anatomical pathology, or perhaps both.

The department itself can be divided into two major sections, a clinical pathology division and an anatomical pathology section. The clinical laboratory and pathology services fall into two areas: (1) those performed directly by the pathologist and (2) those performed under the pathologist's responsibility and supervision but actually conducted by a medical technologist.

It is the pathologist's role to examine all surgical specimens (including autopsies, frozen sections, and tissue consultations). Under the pathologist's supervision, a medical technologist's functions fall into these areas: (1) bacteriology, (2) biochemistry, (3) blood bank, (4) hematology, (5) tissue preparation, (6) organ banks which certain hospitals have to store human organs and tissues used in transplant surgery (for example, corneas and kidneys), and may include (7) nuclear medicine and isotopes.

Some hospitals may contract with private laboratories outside the hospital known as reference labs.

Staffing

The majority of employees in the clinical laboratories are registered medical technologists or medical laboratory technicians. A registered technologist must complete a bachelor's degree in an accredited college or university studying specified science courses in a school of medical technology approved by the Council on Medical Education and the Hospitals of the American Medical Association. The technologist must then pass an examination given by the American Society of Clinical Pathologists (ASCP).

Other personnel working in the clinical laboratory include blood bank technologists, certified laboratory assistants, cytotechnologists, histotechnologists, and microbiologists.

There may be some non-registered personnel working in the clinical laboratory, since there is a shortage of qualified personnel in certain parts of the country. From time to time, persons with Ph.D. degrees in special science disciplines (such as chemistry) also work in the department.

The number of employees will vary with the workload in the department. Departments that are heavily involved in teaching or research or that handle outside requests will obviously vary in staffing patterns. A specific hospital staffing pattern can only be determined after an on-site analysis is conducted and knowledge of the specific workloads within the hospital is available.

As for the medical technologists themselves, there have been studies that suggest what the average workload for a technologist should be per year. These studies consider the types of tests and indicate the differences between hospitals that have a high, medium, or low volume. A staffing and workload analysis is critical when one determines how much space and equipment is needed to run a proper laboratory operation. Government studies show that most hospital laboratories have been showing annual workload increases of approximately 10 percent,[1] which indicates that the workload will be doubled in approximately nine years. This explosion of testing has caused severe expansion problems for hospital laboratories. However, experience with improved techniques in automation suggests that a greater volume of work can be done in the same work area, depending on the clinical laboratory involved.

Location and Physical Facilities

Laboratory facilities may be located either on the ground floor or the first floor. The first floor offers easy accessibility to the outpatients who are sent to the laboratory. It is not as important for inpatients to come to this area, since much of the laboratory's work (that is, collecting specimens) is done on the nursing units.

In determining the overall size of the laboratory, it is important that consideration be give to each functional technical unit—that is, microbiology, chemistry, hematology, and pathology. Only after the size of each individual unit has been established can architectural layouts be properly constructed to fit into the complete program of the laboratory department. The square-foot-per-patient-bed ratio is no longer considered an adequate guide for determining the size of a laboratory. Any plans for a laboratory should be based on work volumes within specific ranges within the laboratory itself. For example, 40,000 to 75,000 tests equates to so many square feet. Since most of the hospitals in this country have between 150 and 200 beds, a typical plan for such a size hospital is shown in Figure 11-1. It includes separate work units for all technical sections—hematology, urinalysis, biochemistry, histology, serology, and bacteriology. Special support areas for glass washing and sterilizing are also available. The pathologist's office and the secretarial/reception area are in a separate cubicle. Also, the laboratory may have a dummy elevator system or special shoots so that laboratory specimens may be received directly from nursing units.

Laboratory Information Systems

It is essential that test results be placed in a report format and promptly and accurately provided to the physicians and health professionals who need to know the results. Traditionally laboratories have manually handled record keeping and reports.

With the growing demand for laboratories to handle more patients and process their test results faster and more efficiently, many hospitals today use automated laboratory information systems. An automated system has the ability to provide quick test ordering, test tracking, and test result reporting. Laboratory data can be presented in a more orderly and timely manner. Physicians, nurses, medical technologists, and other allied health professionals have access to test results as soon as tests are completed. Other benefits include reduced reporting errors and improved legibility.

Automated information systems may also be used to gather statistics on physician ordering and to study certain susceptibilities in patients in order to optimize drug dosages as prescribed by physicians.

In addition to the benefits of increased speed and accuracy in reporting results, automated systems are also used to create anatomic pathology reports, to report on quality control, and to maintain inventory records.

Laboratory Quality Review

In addition to JCAHO's quality review of hospitals, the College of American Pathologists (CAP) has its own quality review program for laboratories known as Q-Probes. Quality in the laboratory not only includes accuracy and precision but also the quick reporting of results to patients. The CAP collects data about blood utilization and cost utilization, analyzes the lab's performance, and sends a report to the laboratory along with the aggregate performance of other labs. Hospitals are able to review lab performance with respect to turnaround time, reporting errors, and nosocomial infection rates and compare it with other laboratories.

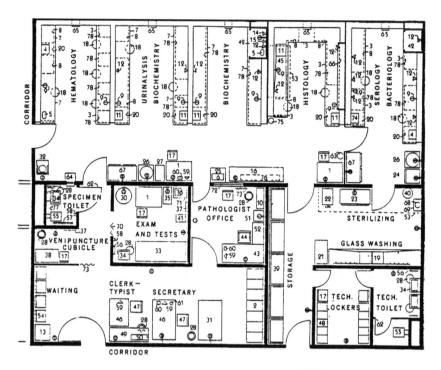

Figure 11-1 Floor Plan for Typical 150–200 Bed Hospital Clinical Laboratory. *Source:* Reprinted from *Planning the Laboratory for the General Hospital*, U.S. D.H.H.S., p. 4, 1961.

Summary

The hospital clinical laboratory has become an essential element in the care of the patient within the hospital. Laboratory tests and examinations are growing rapidly in number and complexity. Since diagnosis and research in medical care are also extremely broad and intensive, the hospital pathologist becomes a critical element in the care of the patient. On the other hand, much of the testing in the laboratory is of routine nature and has been relegated to sophisticated equipment that can produce numerous tests in a brief period of time.

The pathologist is the spokesperson not only for the ancillary department, but in a way is the conscience of the medical staff. The pathologist's crucial role on the tissue committee involves interpreting and guiding physicians' practices through laboratory procedures and tests. Thus, this department and the pathologist in particular are key elements in the hospital's quality assurance program.

RADIOLOGY DEPARTMENT

If diagnosis is the cornerstone of modern medical medicine, then the radiology department, which may also be referred to as the medical imaging department, is the cornerstone of medical diagnosis. The field of radiology had its beginning on Nov. 8, 1895, when an astute observer and professor of physics at the University of Wurzburg in Bavaria, Wilhelm Röentgen, discovered x-rays. The discovery traveled quickly. Within a matter of weeks, physicists and physicians throughout the world were producing x-rays of various types. They were quickly applied to the practice of medicine.

X-rays, when properly applied, permit a trained physician to recognize many medical conditions not otherwise diagnosable in a living patient. In addition, radiation beams, carefully administered in sufficient doses have been found to be an effective treatment method for many diseases. These beams, emitted from x-ray tubes, gave birth to such devices as datatrons and cyclatrons, which are so important in therapeutic radiology. This led to a separate discipline called radiation therapy or radiotherapy. High energy machines such as linear accelerators, employing high particle acceleration, are also used in radiotherapy. Today, considerable progress is being made toward further use of diagnostic and therapeutic radiation procedures.

Functions

The principal functions of the radiology (x-ray) department are to assist the physicians and other health team members in the diagnosis and therapy of a patient's disease through the use of radiography, fluoroscopy, and radioisotopes. There are several special procedures or diagnostic methods used in a modern hospital x-ray department. Fluoroscopy is a means by which body structures are viewed by sending x-rays through the body part to be examined and then observing the shadows cast on a fluorescent (glowing) screen. Cineradiography is a means of converting the fluorescent screen images into radiographs or even into motion pictures. Stereoscopy is the method of taking two radiographs from slightly different angles, thereby allowing physicians to view the body structure in three dimensions.

Advances in imaging as a result of computerization have led to the utilization of high-tech methods in the radiology department. One of the first applications of x-rays and computers was computerized axial tomography (CAT). In the CAT method, a carriage is rotated, allowing an x-ray team to scan a narrow cross section of the body. Many such scans are taken—perhaps as many as 180—at very small distances from each other. These images are then collected and displayed with the use of a computer. While an x-ray can only scan a fractured or broken bone, a CAT scan can also reveal infection and bleeding. Some computerized tomography utilizes three-dimensional imaging, capable of rotating images to give different views of various tissues.

While computerized tomography uses radiation to create an image, magnetic resonance imaging (MRI) can expose internal anatomy without using ionizing radiation. The machinery used resembles a tunnel in which the patient lies. Intensive magnetic force causes the protons found in the molecules of the body to spin and align according to patients. This proton movement gives off energy signals which are measured by radio frequency and assembled into clear photographic images of cross sections of the body. The MRI is able to produce pictures which show changes in bone marrow and the stages of hemorrhage. Tumors, tendons, ligaments, and cartilage also show up more clearly in MRI.

Both computerized axial tomography and magnetic resonance imaging can only show the structural makeup of tissue. There is a newer imaging method called positron emission tomography (PET) that is capable of providing three-dimensional metabolic and functional views of organs. The equipment used is called a cyclotron. It generates radioisotopes to produce cross-sectional images of the body. PET is particularly valuable in the diagnosis of coronary artery disease as it allows cardiologists to study cardiac tissue without using invasive procedures like cardiac catheterization. Also, PET has been utilized to diagnose stroke, brain tumors, epilepsy, alzheimer's disease, and schizophrenia.

There is another imaging method called ultrasound that uses a doppler technique to scan internal organs. It produces moving shadows on a display screen. Special probes are designed for specific anatomical regions which enable rapid diagnosis of internal organs. Ultrasound has been widely used to visualize a fetus within a mother's womb. Fetal abnormalities can be detected, and the sex of the unborn child can usually be distinguished. Some ultrasound instruments have doppler techniques capable of displaying blood flow and diagnosing cardiac problems.

Nuclear Medicine

In some hospitals, nuclear medicine may be part of the radiology department. Nuclear medicine procedures, like other imaging methods, are valuable techniques in diagnosis and treatment. However, nuclear medicine procedures have the ability to assess tissue function as well as metabolism and blood flow. An imaging agent called radiopharmaceutical is injected into a patient. Radiopharmaceuticals contain a small amount of a radioactive element that attaches itself to organs. Different agents are used to attach to the specific organs under study. A camera records the radioactivity emitted by the organ and surrounding tissue, and a planar image is produced. Nuclear medicine has a technology similar to computerized tomography called single photon emission computed tomography (SPECT). Like CAT scans, SPECT produces cross sections of an organ. It can more accurately detect heart and brain abnormalities than other nuclear medicine procedures. SPECT also has growing potential in evaluating bone disorders and detecting tumors, trauma, and infection.

Radiation Therapy

A form of ancillary service related to the x-ray or medical imaging is radiation therapy. Radiation therapy is a form of treatment used in the control of localized cancers. This service is generally found in larger hospitals and regional medical centers. Traditional x-ray equipment uses x-rays or roentgen rays that are applied to electromagnetic, nonparticulate, ionizing what are produced by manmade machines. In radiation therapy, the radiations are either naturally occurring or artificially produced from radioactive elements. The equipment used may include a linear (electron) accelerator or a similar device called a betatron. This equipment generates high-energy radiations. Patients undergoing radiation therapy usually receive small doses several times a week for a period of four to seven weeks. This service may be the responsibility of the hospital radiologist, but often there is a separate clinical department of radiation therapy headed by a physician trained in that specialty.

The radiology department is also responsible for invasive procedures. There is a commonly used procedure called angiography, which is the technique of using a contrast medium and injecting it into the patient's blood vessel, thereby allowing the blood supply (with the contrast medium) to reveal the structure and state of health of the organ.

A secondary mission of the radiology department is to engage in essential research for medical advancement and to participate in educational and inservice programs for hospital residents and the medical staff. Finally, the hospital might be involved in the training of radiologic technologists and other x-ray technical specialists.

Organization

In large hospitals, the radiology department may be organized into three separate sections: diagnostic radiology, therapeutic radiology, and nuclear medicine. In small hospitals, these may be arranged in one organization. The department is under the general direction and supervision of a competent radiologist, a graduate of a medical school who is licensed to practice in the state. This person is appointed as a member of the medical staff and should have considerable specialized training in radiology, either diagnostic or therapeutic or both, and be certified by the American Board of Radiology. Radiation therapists are certified by the American Board of Radiology. Frequently, the radiologist supervises a person called the chief x-ray technician. The radiologist is the clinical department head and accordingly has all the medical-administrative responsibilities that go with that position. In the larger context, the radiologist, as administrator of the department, is responsible to the administrator of the hospital; as a specialist concerned with the quality of care, the radiologist is responsible to the medical staff. Members of the medical staff send their patients to the department for diagnosis and treatment. The outpatient services account for approximately 50 percent of all the x-ray work, including that from the emergency department. The various inpatient nursing units also send patients to the department for procedures during the working day.

Location and Physical Facilities

The x-ray department, or at least a portion of it, should be located on the first floor of the hospital in order to be conveniently accessible to outpatients and inpatients scheduled for admission. If possible, it is preferable to locate the x-ray department close to elevators and adjoining the outpatient department. It is best to locate the department in a wing of the hospital with the x-ray rooms at the extreme end of the wing. In such a configuration, the traffic pattern through the department will be minimized, and less shielding from the x-rays will be required due to the exterior walls around the x-ray rooms.

A well-planned, x-ray diagnostic department will ensure an efficient flow of service, allowing patients to be scheduled properly and expediently with a minimum of movement and distance for both the x-ray staff and the patients. The number of x-ray machines to be installed in the unit will depend, of course, on the size of the hospital, the number of beds in the hospital, and the needs of the community that the hospital services.

Flexibility in the design of the department is important, particularly in a smaller hospital. It is a prerequisite for the handling of a potential increase in the workload and volume. If sufficient space is allocated to begin with, an increase in volume can be handled quite easily by adding additional staff members and installing another machine. When designing and planning a radiology department, or reviewing whether a radiology department should be expanded, procedure standards for room utilization are extremely helpful. There may be individual variations due to the complexity of the examination mix; however, there are guidelines that can be used in determining the number of examination rooms necessary in the x-ray suite. One figure shows that approximately 6,000 examinations per room per year is average.[2] A typical layout for a diagnostic x-ray suite for a 150- to 200-bed hospital is shown in Figure 11-2.

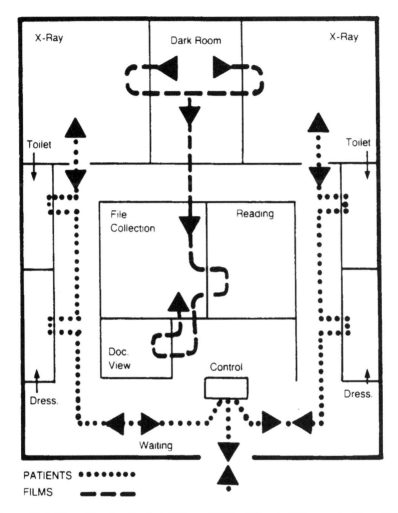

Figure 11-2 Floor Plan for Typical 150- to 200-Bed Hospital Diagnostic X-ray Suite. *Source:* Reprinted from *Diagnostic X-Ray Suites for the General Hospital*, U.S. D.H.H.S., p. 2, 1959.

Staffing

The basic employee in the radiology department is the radiologic technologist or x-ray technician. There must be a sufficient number of these employees in the department to respond to the patients' needs. These technologists should be trained in x-ray work and should be eligible for membership in the American Society of Radiologic Technologists. Technicians perform their work under the supervision of the radiologist and usually a chief technician. The number of technicians required will vary between two and three depending on the workload (volume) and the value of the cases. Factors to be considered are the patients' status (whether or not they are ambulatory) and whether the technicians transport the patients themselves. Technologists must be additionally trained to operate the commonly used high-tech imaging methods.

FREESTANDING IMAGING CENTERS

Today a growing number of hospitals are providing similar diagnostic and therapeutic radiological procedures that they offer in their radiology departments in outpatient centers separate from the hospital. These centers are referred to as freestanding imaging centers. The advantages of freestanding imaging centers include: more favorable reimbursements for outpatient procedures than inpatient procedures; a patient referral source for the hospital; and more convenience to the patient.

Some hospitals are also involved in mobile diagnostic and therapeutic radiologic procedures. They offer radiological services on wheels as a way to take these services to patients at other hospitals or at work sites.

ANESTHESIOLOGY DEPARTMENT

The development of anesthesia began with the introduction of ether by Dr. Morton in 1847. Unlike the development of anesthesia in Great Britain, the practice of anesthesia in the United States was not always a strictly medical discipline. Though there were some surgeons who became interested in the problems of anesthesia, these represented only a minority. It was not until the 1930s, when the study of the physiology of trauma in surgery began to unfold, that physicians became acutely interested in the discipline of anesthesiology. Prior to that time, nurse anesthetists were primarily involved in the giving of anesthesia. The Association of Nurse Anesthetists was formed in 1931. Since that time, the association has been a significant force in improving the standards for the training and education of nurse anesthetists. Anesthesia received a great boost during World War II, when many of the physicians in the military, particularly in the army, were given training in anesthesia before being sent to the hospitals to work. A nurse anesthetist is a registered professional nurse who has been trained in the administration of anesthesia. The nurse anesthetist may also assist patients with respiratory or cardiopulmonary conditions. After finishing the education and being certified, the individual may use the initials CRNA (Certified Registered Nurse Anesthetist) after his or her name.

There has been dramatic growth in the discipline of anesthesia. In 1940, there were approximately 38 hospitals offering residency programs in anesthesiology.[3] In the same year, there were only 105 board-certified anesthesiologists. Today, anesthesiology is the sixth-largest specialty group in the country. There are 17,000 members of whom 8,172 are Fellows of the American College of Anesthesiologists.[4]

Functions

The anesthesiology department has three main functions: (1) to render a patient insensible to pain during a surgical procedure, (2) to control the patient's physiology during the procedure and to follow the patient during the immediate postoperative period, and (3) to manage and supervise the therapy by inhalation of gaseous substances. The anesthesia department is also responsible for providing local or block anesthesia in certain surgical procedures and diseases.

Hospital administrators, nurses, physicians, and anesthesiologists all must be aware that patients going to surgery have to sign certain permission slips (informed consent for surgery) prior to surgery. A patient must be informed about the surgical procedure and the liabilities and risks involved before signing the permit to undergo the procedure. It is also the anesthesiologist's responsibility to visit the patient prior to surgery. The patient should be informed about the anesthesia that will be used, how it will be administered, and what that patient may feel.

Anesthesiologists also have a role in caring for the critical or intensive care patients. They may function as primary care physicians, cooperate with primary care physicians, or act as consulting physicians. Anesthesiologists are involved with patients' dietary management and patients' problems regarding respiratory and circulatory insufficiency.

Organization

Most hospitals have a separate department of anesthesiology. Those hospitals that do not have a separate department usually include anesthesia as a function of the department of surgery. Most often, the department of anesthesiology is headed by a physician who is trained in the medical discipline of anesthesia and, hopefully, is board certified. The department frequently has more than one physician anesthesiologist. It is quite common to have nurse anesthetists in the department. Both the physician specialist and the nurse anesthetist administer anesthesia. When a physician anesthesiologist is not available, for example, some rural hospitals may use nurse anesthetists exclusively to administer anesthesia. The responsibility for this department is then delegated to either the chief of surgery or to another designated person. In such cases, the operating surgeon is responsible for the professional acts of the nurse anesthetists.

Location and Physical Facilities

The Anesthesiology Department is usually near the hospital's operating suite. A typical layout for an operating room is shown in Figure 11-3.

Staffing

The precise number of physician anesthetists and nurse anesthetists employed in a given hospital will depend upon the number and types of surgical procedures and the number of obstetrical deliveries in the hospital. Personnel in the anesthesia department are required to be on call; this, of course, has an impact on staffing patterns. The nurse anesthetists, depending on the contractual arrangement between the anesthesiologist and the hospital, either work directly for the anesthesiologist or are hospital employees. In any event, the nurse anesthetists function under the technical supervision of the anesthesiologist.

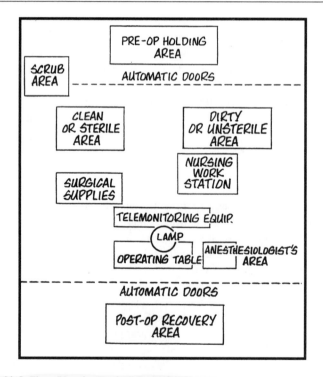

Figure 11-3 Floor Plan for Typical Operating Room

NOTES

1. U.S. Department of Health, Education, and Welfare, Public Health Service, Division of Hospitals and Medical Facilities, *Planning the Laboratory for the General Hospital,* p. 30.

2. Hospital Survey Committee, *Utilization of Facilities for Diagnostic Radiology* (Philadelphia, Pa.: Hospital Survey Committee, 1975), p. 79.

3. *1990-1991 Directory of Graduate Medical Education Programs,* (Chicago, Ill.: American Medical Association, 1990).

4. "The Diamond Jubilee," The American Society of Anesthesiologists, Inc., 1980, p. 22.

Chapter 12

Other Ancillary Services

Key Terms

Pulmonary function studies • Ventilators • Electroencephalography •
Electrocardiography • Physician therapist • Occupational therapist •
Comprehensive outpatient rehabilitative facility (CORF) • Decentralized
pharmacy • Formulary unit dose system • Floor stock • Narcotic drugs •
Food and Drug Administration (FDA)

RESPIRATORY CARE DEPARTMENT

A discipline closely related to anesthesiology is respiratory therapy. The respiratory care field has developed rapidly under the sponsorship of such organizations as the American College of Physicians and the American Society of Anesthesiologists. In today's hospital, respiratory therapy is an extremely important facet in the diagnosis and treatment of certain categories of patients. The Respiratory Care Department at one time was known as the inhalation therapy department. The older term referred to the treatment of patients with the use of oxygen and other inhalation therapies.

The Respiratory Care Department embodies the therapeutic value of oxygen and other therapies together with, among the newer studies and techniques, pulmonary function studies and blood gas analysis. The respiratory therapy department is involved in both diagnostic and therapeutic treatment of inpatients and outpatients. The department is particularly important in the treatment and diagnosis of patients with pulmonary disease and certain cardiac ailments. It is responsible for administering breathing treatments such as bronchodilator therapies to patients, setting up equipment for oxygen administration, giving chest physiotherapy to patients, and managing the adequate functioning of ventilators. The respiratory department also participates in cardiac arrest codes by providing all the equipment and supplies needed to assist the patient with ventilation. All procedures given to the patients are performed either by a physician or a trained respiratory therapist. These procedures can be administered to the patient only upon the prescribed written orders of a physician.

ELECTROENCEPHALOGRAPHY

One of the more specialized ancillary services in hospitals is the electroencephalography (EEG) testing service. This is generally part of the neurosurgery or neurology section of the hospital or medical staff. This service is an indispensable tool for solving neurosurgical or neurological problems. The EEG test measures the electrical brain activity of the patient. It is frequently used when patients have suffered serious head injuries; in such circumstances, an EEG test can be a lifesaver. The EEG testing was formerly used primarily for the diagnosis of seizures and the detection of tumors. However, in recent years the EEG test has been utilized in analyzing many problems, from fainting and mild headaches to epileptic disorders and severe trauma from a head injury. The test is conducted by highly trained technicians upon a physician's order. The EEG test has to be conducted in a room where extraneous noise cannot be picked up. If the room is not perfectly situated, certain artifacts will appear on the EEG readout and make it worthless. The EEG laboratory does not have a high volume, like laboratory and x-ray. Frequently, however, EEG lab technicians are on 24-hour call for emergency determinations. The EEG tests are used in determining both the first signs of life and the last signs of life coming from the brain. Often the EEG test can be the means of determining whether the patient is legally alive or dead.

There are hybrids of the EEG technique that include studies when the patient is asleep or partially asleep. The sleep EEGs are particularly important in the study of different types of epilepsy. With the advent of CAT Scanners, some people believe that EEGs have lost some of their value. However, the EEG printouts continue to be used; rather than the brain scan replacing this ancillary study, the EEG test is frequently used in combination with the brain scan.

Recently, the diagnostic role of electroencephalography has been expanded to include a therapeutic one, too. This has been illustrated by the utilization of EEGs in sleep disorder clinics to treat patients with problems such as sleep apnea.

HEART STATION

Cardiac diagnostic services are usually provided in the area of the hospital commonly referred to as the heart station. One of the core products of the heart station is electrocardiography (EKG).

The EKG is used most frequently on patients having cardiac disease, suspected cardiac disease, or complications of cardiac disease. It is also useful as a chest baseline test prior to surgery. If an electrocardiogram is abnormal, detailed information regarding the diagnosis and management of the patient is provided; this makes the course of the patient's treatment much more reasonable and scientific. An electrocardiogram is taken with special equipment to produce an electrocardiograph. The basic EKG machine is a table-type of apparatus on wheels that is rolled to the inpatient's bedside. It is operated by highly skilled technicians.

The interpreter of the cardiogram is usually a cardiologist or an internist who is skilled in reading electrocardiogram tracings. The technician must be trained to take multilead tracings, that is, tracings from the 12 leads that are normally attached to the patient to obtain a standard electrocardiogram.

Hospitals may use a three-channel EKG cart with computerized printout attachments as part of their equipment. In this arrangement, the technician goes to the patient's bedside with an electrocardiograph cart that has a telephone receiver attached. The tracings may be sent over the telephone lines to be read. The reading is then relayed to a computer that interprets the reading and prints out at the patient's bedside within 20 to 50 seconds what is called an "unconfirmed" electrocardiograph reading. It is unconfirmed because the computer has read it, not a cardiologist. The unconfirmed reading is usually confirmed by having a hospital cardiologist "overread" the computerized interpretation printout. The physician who reads the printout signs it as if the technician in the hospital had taken the tracing. The advantages of the shared computerized electrocardiogram system are basically two: (1) it provides a high degree of consistency and quality, and (2) it provides fast feedback time on the readings.

Though the basic electrocardiogram is the most common service in hospitals, there are variations of electrocardiograph tracings that are done for different purposes to determine the special diagnostic problem. For example, stress testing or treadmill exercise testing is a procedure in which a patient is placed under severe stress, and the patient's heart impulses are then interpreted in those conditions. There is also echoencephalography and Holter monitoring, procedures in which a patient wears a tracing or monitoring device while active for a period of hours; tracings are then made and interpreted usually through a computer reading.

Nuclear medicine procedures such as a multigated acquisition (MUGA) wall motion study and thallium spect and planar tests are also used to evaluate patients with coronary artery disease, chest pain, and questionable EKG and stress tests. Other diagnostic testing provided by the heart station includes echocardiography, doppler modalities, and peripheral vascular studies. The heart station is responsible for pacemaker insertion and evaluation.

REHABILITATIVE MEDICINE

The discipline of physical medicine and rehabilitation is a medical specialty concerned with the diagnosis and treatment of certain musculoskeletal defects and neuromuscular diseases and problems. Physical medicine began to emerge during World War I when the Army was involved in vocational guidance and training programs for the disabled. However, it was not until some time following World War II that the specialty became well known and formal training programs became more available.

The first three-year residency in physical medicine and rehabilitation was established at the Mayo Clinic. Today, there are a growing number of hospitals specializing in complete physical medicine and rehabilitation services. A physical medicine department is headed by a physician called a physiatrist whose special interests lie in physical medicine and rehabilitation. The financial arrangements between the physiatrist and the hospital management are usually on a simplified salaried or "fee-for-service" basis. Fee-for-service is a method whereby a physician bills the patient or third party for each physician service rendered.

Areas of rehabilitative medicine include physical therapy, occupational therapy, and speech therapy. Physical therapy is commonly prescribed by physicians, and the referred patient is evaluated and treated by the physical therapist. These professionals have earned either a bachelor's, master's, or doctoral degree in physical therapy, or they have a postbaccalaureate certificate of training. The physical therapists are licensed by the individual state and are referred to as PTs. The therapist uses light, heat, water, electricity, ultrasound, and physical and mechanical force to treat the patient's illness or pain.

Although physical facilities will vary widely, hospitals will usually have a large room or gymnasium for physical therapy. In this area there will be sufficient space for patient cubicles, dressing rooms, toilets and showers, running water, and a great deal of physical therapy equipment. This equipment may include diathermy units, ultrasound devices, gym mats, Hubbard tanks, parallel walking bars, ultraviolet lamps, whirlpool baths, exercising steps, progressive resistance apparatus, and treatment tables.

Hospitals may offer occupational therapy services under the direction of a physician. The occupational therapist is involved in treating physical disability and in teaching the patient compensatory techniques to perform daily activities, frequently with the assistance of self-help aids. The occupational therapist is also involved in perceptual testing and training. The therapist is guided by the physician when creating certain educational and functional activities to help patients. Like the physical therapist, the occupational therapist has earned either a bachelor's, master's, or doctoral degree and may be registered.

Finally, speech therapy has become more common in community hospitals. This is a therapeutic discipline that uses speech therapists and physicians to correct a patient's speech defects or to reeducate the patient who may have lost the power of speech through disease, accident, or stroke. Often the speech therapists are involved in stressing methods to correct speech and language deficits with the objective of bringing patients back as close as possible to normal speech functions. The speech therapist also has earned either a bachelor's, master's, or doctoral degree and may be registered.

Medicare has approved the concept of outpatient rehabilitative medicine by permitting hospitals to set up comprehensive outpatient rehabilitation facilities (CORFs). A CORF is a non-residential facility that is established to provide diagnostic, therapeutic, and restorative services. Services are provided at a single, fixed location, by or under the supervision of a physician. The services include physical therapy, occupational therapy, and speech therapy, as well as supportive service in psychology, social services, and orthotics/prosthetics.

THE PHARMACY

The hospital pharmacy has the role of manufacturing, compounding, and dispensing drugs and other diagnostic and therapeutic chemical substances that are used in the hospital. Smaller hospitals may not have a regular pharmacy department; they may purchase items from a local pharmacist and maintain only a limited supply under lock and key. In most hospitals, a full-time pharmacist is available, sometimes with several assistants.

Some hospitals may have a decentralized pharmacy system whereby there is one main pharmacy and satellite pharmacies on each nursing unit of the hospital. Some hospitals may also have outpatient pharmacies.

The pharmacy may sell items to the general public in addition to the patients, but this practice is generally discouraged by administrators. Whether the pharmacy department manufactures certain solutions or drugs is a matter of hospital policy. For quality and economy reasons, most hospitals prefer to purchase the drugs and solutions already made, whether they be for injections or for intravenous administration.

The pharmacist who heads the department must have completed a five-year program in an accredited school of pharmacy and must be licensed. Some pharmacists pursue a doctor of pharmacy degree (Pharm.D.) Pharmacy technicians function to assist the pharmacist in prepackaging drugs, controlling inventory, distributing floor stock items, and assisting in activities not requiring professional judgment. Pharmacy technicians may be trained on the job or in a hospital-based program.

Pharmacy and Therapeutics Committee

The pharmacy and therapeutics committee functions as a liaison between the pharmacy and medical staff with the role of overseeing the medical aspects of the hospital's pharmacy activities. Members usually include physicians, a pharmacist, a nurse, and an administrator. Though the pharmacy and therapeutics committee recommends the standard drugs to be dispensed in the hospital, it is the pharmacist's responsibility in the vast majority of hospitals to select the brand or supplier of drug dispensed for all medication orders and prescriptions, unless a specific notation to the contrary is made by the prescriber.

A key duty of the pharmacy and the therapeutics committee is to develop a formulary of acceptable drugs. The formulary contains a list of drugs, usually by generic names, approved and available for use within the hospital. Recommended dosages, contraindications, warnings, and pharmacology are described in the formulary. Other functions of the committee include educating the professional staff, reviewing drug reactions and studies, participating in quality assurance, and establishing cost effective drug therapy.

Drug Distribution System

Once the hospital or pharmacy receives the drugs and supplies, they must be distributed. Distribution is primarily to the nursing units where inpatients receive the majority of the drugs dispensed by the pharmacy. Generally the drugs fall into one of three categories:

1. Items sent to the nursing units for floor stock inventory. These are items regularly stored in the unit and not charged to the patients directly. Examples of such nonchargeable items are rubbing compounds and antiseptics for wounds and bandages.
2. Patient-chargeable stock items kept in the nursing unit. These include disposable enemas and other disposable external preparations.
3. Common prescription drugs that are dispensed and charged only upon the receipts of a prescription by a physician. This category of prescription drugs represents the vast majority of drugs used and also represents the greatest cost in the pharmacy.

A common method of dispensing medication to patients is the unit dose system. The pharmacy either packages the medication or receives from vendors prepackaged medications in specific dosages. The latter method allows for better control and less waste of the drug; on the other hand, there is with this method the additional cost of packaging the drugs. Under the unit dose system, a 24-hour supply of medications is dispensed to each nursing unit. The medications are kept in patient drawers in the nursing unit's medication cart. The drawers are combined into cassettes, and cassettes are exchanged by the pharmacy at a designated time every day. The unit dose system offers greater convenience to the hospital pharmacist, the nurses, and the patients. With this system, there is increased efficiency of operations, and preparation and distribution errors are reduced.

The pharmacy department is also responsible for the preparation and distribution of intravenous fluid (IV) solutions or parental feeding products like nutritional substances and also chemotherapeutic agents. The timing of preparation and delivery is crucial, since some solutions are stable for only a given time. A sterile environment is necessary for drug preparation, therefore laminar flow hoods are needed for the pharmacy department preparing such solutions.

Control of Narcotics and Barbiturates

The hospital must exercise strict control over the dispensing of narcotics and barbiturates. These drugs must be kept under security both in the pharmacy and in the nursing units. Thorough and adequate records must be kept on narcotics and barbiturates. At the change of each nursing shift, a narcotics and barbiturates count is taken. Maintenance of narcotics in the hospital must be in conformance with the Harrison Drug Act and the Food, Drug, and Cosmetic Act for Barbiturates. Physicians must note their narcotic license number on the prescription when they order a narcotic. When they give a telephone order for narcotics to a nurse, they generally must place their written signature and number on the patient's medical record within 48 hours. Most hospitals have instituted a procedure by which narcotic orders must be reordered by the physician after a certain length of time. A definition of narcotic drugs is provided in the Comprehensive Drug Abuse Prevention and Control Act of 1970.

Generic versus Brand Name Drugs

The federal government and other agencies are encouraging the use of generic drugs because the cost for the generic drug is considerably below that of brand names. A drug's generic name is the official (nonproprietary) name by which the drug is scientifically known, based on its chemical substance irrespective of the manufacturer. A drug's brand name or trade name is the registered trademark given to the drug by its manufacturer. An industry report showed that direct sales reached 33.2 billion and of that amount 8.3 billion, or 25 percent, was for generic prescription drugs and 24.9 billion for brand name drugs.[1]

Selling Drugs to Hospitals

A discussion about hospital pharmacies and the sale of drugs would not be complete without mention of the drug "detail men" or pharmaceutical service representatives who are hired by the major drug manufacturing companies. These individuals provide a valuable service, particularly to the physicians who order the drugs. The detail men acquaint physicians in the hospital with new drugs and try to reinforce the use of existing drugs. Hospitals buy the vast majority of their drugs through group purchasing arrangements where hospitals group together to purchase items to receive volume discounts. More than 97 percent of all hospitals are involved in some type of group purchasing arrangement through which they can buy their drugs and supplies.[2] The dollar volume spent by hospitals on drugs continues to increase annually.[3] The purchase of drugs has been increasing between 5 and 12 percent a year. Since 1976, there has been a 400 percent increase in the dollars that hospitals spend. Hospitals typically spend 8 to 12 percent of their total inpatient cost on drugs. This is expected to increase over the next several years.[4]

Quality Assurance

A hospital's quality assurance program for pharmaceutical services must establish policies and procedures for the preparation and distribution of drugs and parental products. The pharmacist should be active in developing criteria and standards for the use of drugs in the hospital. Drug misuse needs to be identified, and corrective measures need to be proposed.

One of the specific tasks accomplished in quality assurance programs is to have drug usage identified according to drug type. Statistics can be developed to indicate what percentage of patients receive certain types of drugs during hospitalization. Another function that the program looks into is drug usage according to diagnosis. Patient diagnoses can be reviewed to determine if any drugs are being used in the presence of a medical problem where there is contraindication for its use, for example, steroids being used in the presence of a peptic ulcer.

On a macro level, the government is also involved in the regulation of pharmaceutical products. According to the Food, Drug and Cosmetic Act of 1906, the Food and Drug Administration (FDA) must ensure the purity of drugs manufactured and sold. The act was amended in 1962 to also include proving the safety of medications.

NOTES

1. The Generic Pharmacy Industry Association, 1989.
2. Stephanie Crawford, *ASHP National Survey of Hospital-Based Pharmaceutical Services—1990,* American Journal of Hospital Pharmacy, Vol. 47, December 1990.

3. 1989 Lilly Hospital Survey, American Journal of Hospital Pharmacy, Vol. 46, November 1989.

4. Quoted from Stephen Schrodelmeyer, Pharm.D., Ph.D., Professor of Pharmaceutical Economics, College of Pharmacy, Univ. of Minnesota, Minneapolis, Minn.

Part VI

Behind the Scenes

Chapter 13

Patient Support Services

Key Terms

American Dietetic Association • Dietitian • Patient menus • Conventional system • Convenience food • Cool • Chill system • Special diets • Contract services • Social worker • Discharge planning • Chaplain • Patient transportation • Patient representative

WHAT ARE SUPPORT SERVICES?

Hospital support services are defined as those hospital departments or cost centers that are not medical ancillary departments. These services do not typically generate patient revenue and are not under the professional direction of a physician as required by JCAHO. There are three types of support services in a hospital: the patient support service departments, the facilities support service departments, and the administrative support service departments. The patient support services may have direct patient contact and include the following areas or departments: dietary, social services, pastoral care, patient escort, and patient ombudsman or patient representative services. The facilities support services include the traditional plant operation services such as environment (housekeeping) services, maintenance, the physical plant, and clinical (biomedical) engineering department. The administrative support services are those nonpatient care departments that directly support the administrative mission of the hospital and include the materials management, human resources, volunteers, and telecommunications departments.

DIETARY DEPARTMENT

No department in the hospital reaches more patients, hospital staff, and visitors than the dietary department. If the food service is efficient and effective, it usually receives only faint praise from patients and personnel. If the food service is perceived inadequate, criticisms abound. Complaining patients often say, "For what I am paying for this room, you would think that the food would be better," "It should be hot," "I could have it when I want it if I were in a hotel," "I should be able to get it at any time." These comments speak to the crucial public relations aspect of the dietary department.

In earlier times, the preparation and delivery of food were under the auspices of the nursing department, the head housekeeper, or the chief cook. Then the housekeeping department underwent an evolution, and the dietary department started to take on a separate entity and the food service was removed from the nursing department. Developments in the world of nutrition and dietetics had an impact on the formation of special dietary departments. The medical profession began to look at the role of proper diet and nutrition as an aid to maintaining good health. A second development was in the evolution of the dietetic profession itself. The dietetic profession, through its membership in the American Dietetic Association, numbers over 16,000 people.[1] The American Dietetic Association has given emphasis to the sophisticated training of dieticians. The association prescribes a dietetic internship as one route to membership of one year of supervised work experience. Dieticians must have earned a bachelor's degree and sometimes a master's degree.

The dietary department has a role in the therapeutic care of the patients as well as in providing standard food menus for the patients and staff. Dieticians plan and direct the food and meal service and teach patients about proper nutrition. Every hospital should have a qualified professional dietician.

Patient Menus

It is the dietician's responsibility to plan menus for the patients and staff. The hospital dietician must have sound technical knowledge about foods as well as sufficient imagination to group foods attractively for meals. Dieticians must be sensitive to the psychological impact that food can have on the well-being of patients. In the past, hospitals were known as institutions serving questionable quality of food, but today's hospitals find themselves catering more to the patients' needs and wants, as well as to their nutritional needs. They offer a selection of meats, vegetables, and desserts, including out-of-season products and hothouse fruits. Many hospitals offer gourmet menus.

Dieticians prefer two- or three-week schedules in preparing their menus. Basic outlines are used, and daily adjustments are made to handle special diet needs. The selective menu (allowing patients more than one food choice) in hospitals has gained wide acceptance and use. As might be expected, the selective menu is easier to implement in the larger hospitals. Menus are modified by having the dietician regularly visit the patients to determine their needs and wants. The public relations aspect of a dietician's visit cannot be underestimated. Improving the nutritional services by reducing patient complaints and making the patients feel they are special, as they should be, is a crucial part of the hospital dietician's role.

Special Diets

There is an increasing use of special diets for hospital patients. This has occurred because of advances in diet therapy and a greater understanding of nutrition. Special diets are actually based on physicians' therapeutic orders that are placed in the patient's medical records. A physician, in consultation with the dietician will recommend a specific diet based on a patient's condition. Special diets for patients are prepared under the direct supervision of a responsible dietician or nutritionist. Since the variety of food may be greatly reduced, it poses a real psychological challenge for the dietician to make the special tray attractive and eye-appealing. Some examples of special diets are low sodium, low cholesterol, high fiber, restricted calorie, diabetic, clear fluids, full liquids, and pureed food.

Type of Food Service

Because of the increasing pressure on hospital management to contain costs, and because of the demands and wants of patients and the changing state of the art in food service, hospitals have explored a variety of different methods to produce and deliver high-quality meals. There are basically four types or methods in the preparation and delivery of food in hospitals: the conventional system, the convenience food system, the cook-chill system, and the frozen-ready (cook-freeze) system. Food service experts describe the four systems as follows:

> The conventional system is the system which uses a menu prepared from basic ingredients daily with preparation assembly and finishing accomplished on the premises.
> The convenience system is the system which used menu items that for the most part have been commercially prepared off the premises and then have been frozen and/or freeze dried in a form that can be easily prepared on site without the need for anything more complex than simple heating. An example of this type of item is the preplated hospital special-diet meal similar to the TV dinner.
> The cook-chill system is the system which entails the use of on-site prepared products that are not necessarily utilized the day of prepara-

tion; they are flash-chilled, stored in the chill state (about 35 degrees F.), and reheated just prior to service.

The frozen ready (cook-freeze) food system is a system which uses primarily a menu that is mass-produced on site, frozen, and stored in a form that requires only tempering (thawing), and reheating before service.

A hospital may not use one single system. The hospital could select a combination of these four systems for its particular production system. Selection among the four systems is, of course, left to the dietician, food service manager, and to hospital administration. The cost—the operating cost per meal and the annual cost per meal—may vary between the least expensive and the most expensive meal. The food costs in the convenience system tend to be higher, and the conventional system tends to be at a lower cost.

Depending on the method of food production the hospital selects, the tray service to the patients will vary. But essentially there are two basic systems of tray service: the centralized and the decentralized. Many hospitals have modifications of each of these systems, due to the physical layout of the hospital. The bulk food delivery system is really a hybrid of the centralized and decentralized systems.

The centralized system is used by many hospitals because it provides for greater efficiency, economy, and supervision, as well as efficient utilization of personnel time. Patient trays are centrally prepared and checked under central supervision along a conveyor belt, somewhat like an assembly line in an automobile industry. The decentralized system is the oldest method of serving food. In the decentralized system, the food is prepared and placed on the patients' trays in substations of the nursing units. This is a less efficient means than the centralized system. Because each nursing unit needs a separate kitchen for the distribution of food, capital costs are increased. One of the weakest links in the centralized food system may be the act of getting the tray to the patient's bedside. Since the trays are brought to the nursing unit in large carts, the food may lose heat or become less cold in transit.

Physical Facilities

The physical facilities of the food preparation area involve more than just a kitchen. The dietary area must have a method of receiving the foodstuffs. Thus, a receiving area and platform and an administrative area are necessary. In addition, once the food is on the premises, it is important to see that there is clean and appropriate storage. There should be a central storage area, both dry storage and refrigerator storage. Further, the food production area must be close to the storage area to reduce the people cost and the cost of transporting the food to the area. In the food preparation area, there are cooking and baking facilities. Numerous broilers, friers, and ovens should be available. There is also a dishwashing area.

Cafeteria Services

The hospital cafeteria, which provides cafeteria service for the hospital staff, the medical staff, visitors, and even ambulatory hospital patients, is under the jurisdiction of the dietary department. It is usually near the food preparation area, so that service elevators or dumbwaiters can aid in transporting the food from the food preparation area to the cafeteria. Two elements in the cafeteria area are the serving lines and the dining area.

There was a time when hospital cafeterias essentially offered subsidized food as a fringe benefit; this allowed hospitals to rationalize lower salaries. As hospital employees' salaries have become more competitive, hospital cafeteria prices have also risen. Many hospitals operate cafeterias with pitiful profit margin goals. Likewise, cafeteria services have expanded. In addition to serving three hot and cold meals a day, some cafeterias have sandwich grills, snack services, and midnight meal services.

Vending Services

Sometimes, hospitals supplement their hospital cafeteria with food and beverage vending machines. It is frequently the dietary department's responsibility to oversee the hospital's vending operations. Usually these vending services are contracted out, but some hospitals do provide their own vending services.

Catering Services

The dietary department is responsible for catering services. Typically, catering services are for the administration, medical staff, and hospital functions such as community meetings and volunteer affairs. Although these services are labor intensive, they can create positive public relations for the dietary department and the hospital.

Contract Food Services

As hospitals continue to explore different methods of delivering and preparing food, they have also been exploring dietary department contract services. The American Hospital Association defines contract services as "a departmental management contract considered to be a formal agreement between a health care institution and a contractor under which the contractor is to provide the institution various management functions and which may include other services in return for a fee."[2]

An increasing number of hospitals engage outside management for their dietary and food areas, usually relying upon commercial companies for this purpose. The results range from quite satisfactory to unsatisfactory. However, on balance, contract food services can do a satisfactory job. There are pros and cons to hospital food management contract services. Some of the advantages of having an outside contracting service include the use of highly specialized trained personnel from an outside source, thereby reducing the need for hospital personnel and the recruitment of such specialists. Indeed, the outside service may provide specialized personnel that the hospital does not have. Further, the outside management group may reduce costs through improved methods and efficiency. The byproduct of this may be a lower personnel staff in the dietary area, depending on the method of food service selected. This could free up space formerly occupied by food preparation equipment in the hospital and allow room for other departments. It also permits the hospital to review regularly the performance of the outside management firm.

Outside contractors would list, as their advantages, higher productivity, outstanding supervision, increased administrative interest, the provision of advanced equipment products, and research on food systems. They would make the point that outside contractors bring more flexibility to the hospital's changing scene. On the other side of the ledger, there are advantages for the hospital in maintaining its own inhouse services. One advantage is employee loyalty, that is, employees who are paid by the hospital may be more loyal. Moreover, hospitals have found that, with full-time employees of the hospital, a certain scheduling flexibility may be achieved. Also, a spirit of teamwork is generated by having the hospital use its own dietary department and by having its dietary employees work with other departments. Some hospitals would argue that, by having all the employees under their jurisdiction, security will be increased. Still, the proprietary food companies have a definite vested interest in offering their services at competitive prices and have proven themselves to be in many instances as efficient and effective in order to retain the hospital's contract.

Expanded Food Service Programs

Hospitals have been expanding their food service programs beyond traditional patient and employee services. New business lines have been created in response to underutilized services in the dietary department and a desire to generate revenue. Some examples of new food service programs are meals for the homebound, frozen dinners for local and regional markets, take-out delis, Sunday brunches for the public, bakeries, off-campus catering, and meals for nursing home residents.

SOCIAL SERVICE DEPARTMENT

Dr. Malcolm MacEachern, the established father of hospital administration, notes in his classic textbook, *Hospital Organization and Management*, that the nineteenth century British hospital had the equivalent of our social worker, called an "almoner." According to MacEachern, the almoner was the individual who represented the community that dispensed alms. The almoner's chief duty was to prevent the abuse of charity. The almoner was also involved deeply in the social programs of the hospital. MacEachern traces this individual from the moralistic almoners of the Middle Ages, noting that the nineteenth century British counterpart had very little of the true spirit of charity. Apparently, the almoner's chief objective was the offering of aid but with the expenditure of as little money as possible. Whatever the merits of the nineteenth century almoner, this individual appears to have been the forerunner of the present-day social worker in the hospital.

America's first organized social service department in a hospital was formed by Dr. Richard C. Cabot at the Massachusetts General Hospital in 1905. At that time, the social worker was a brand new means of complementing the efforts of physicians in delivering better medical care. Dr. Cabot's projected role for the newly formed profession was "to investigate and report to the doctor domestic and social conditions bearing on diagnosis and treatment, to fill the gap between his orders and their fulfillment, and to form the link between the hospital and the many societies, institutions, and persons whose deed could be enlisted."[3]

Qualifications of a Medical Social Worker

Social workers in the social service departments are highly trained individuals. Specifically, they must have graduated from a baccalaureate program and may have taken advanced training at the master's degree level. The American Association of Medical Social Workers has set down the qualifications of training and eligibility for membership in that organization.

Functions of the Department

The modern-day hospital can expect the social service department to make six specific contributions to the mission of the hospital:

1. to aid the health team to understand the social, economic, and emotional factors that affect the patient's illness, treatment, and recovery
2. to aid the patient, the patient's family, and the hospital staff to understand these factors and to make constructive use of the resources in the medical care system, this is a key part of efficient discharge planning

3. to promote the well-being of the patient and improve the patient's family's morale by working with the family and the patient

4. to improve the mission of the hospital by becoming involved in hospital education and activities with the hospital staff and members of the outside community

5. to offer better patient care by making various services, including those outside the hospital, available to the patient

6. to improve the utilization of the community's resources and to impact these resources in order to aid patient and family needs when the patients leave the hospital.

More specifically, the social service department may also offer adoption assistance, information concerning community resources and support groups, referrals to placement facilities, e.g., nursing homes, home care services, and assistance in acquiring durable medical equipment.

One observer, in analyzing the extent to which the social worker can affect the patient and the patient's recovery, commented:

> The extent to which the patient is ready to accept advice from the social worker is dependent on two points: 1) the degree to which his physician sees the need for advice from the social worker and 2) the patient's understanding of the services of the social workers. They found that the physician's understanding not only of the social and emotional factors in relation to the care of a particular individual, but also his understanding of the functions and skills of the social worker and being of service to his patient, definitely reflects the degree to which the social service department is dependent. The department is used by the physician in the care of his patient. The awareness of the physician of this service is the important criterion in determining the effectiveness of the social services.[4]

The important point is that if social service is truly to be effective, it must be directly related to communication with the physician and the patient.

A New Role for the Medical Social Worker

The social worker has taken on an important role in aiding the process of quality assurance. As a committee member on the quality assurance program of a hospital, the social worker's most important contribution is in the area of discharge planning. JCAHO recommends that the social service department have a written policy and procedure for discharge planning. Discharge planning is the organized, centralized system to ensure that each hospitalized patient has a planned program to provide the needed continuing care and follow up the patient requires. Physicians, nurses, and administrators frequently look to the social worker to aid in arranging programs to enable patients to receive continuing care after they leave the hospital environment.

In order for discharge planning to be effective, it should begin at the time a patient is admitted to the hospital. A crucial aspect of discharge planning is the location of placement facilities such as long-term care facilities and rehabilitation facilities for patients who are unable to go home following their hospitalization. This is a challenging task for the medical social worker. The social worker impacts directly not only on the patient's well-being but also on the cost effectiveness and efficiency of the hospital's operations. If the patient is not moved into a placement facility, the hospital runs a risk of losing money. Thus, willingly or not, the social worker in the hospital environment has become an agent of the administration and the financial manager in saving the hospital money.

Beyond that, the medical social service department may yield benefits that are quite intangible. Though unmeasured in dollars, these benefits are reflected in the comments of the patients and their families that the social workers serve. Hospitals have found that medical social service departments have become an indispensable element in the hospital organization. Physicians frequently add their praise for the medical social worker, indicating their great contribution to the rapid rehabilitation of patients.

Psychiatric Social Worker

There is a specialized role for the social worker who works with patients who have emotional and mental as well as social and personal problems. The psychiatric social worker assists psychiatrists in diagnosis and treatment, helps the patient's family to adjust, and engages in discharge planning activities also.

PASTORAL CARE SERVICES

Chaplains and members of religious orders, e.g., sisters, function in the hospital as active listeners for patients and patients' families and as providers of spiritual support. The hospital chaplain engages in crisis intervention and stress management by helping the patient to discover and use his own strength and faith. Chaplains frequently act as intermediaries between the patient, the family and physicians. Some chaplains take part in interdisciplinary staff meetings, read the patients' clinical charts, and write notes in the patients' medical records.

PATIENT ESCORT SERVICES

The patient escort or transport department provides transportation either by wheelchair or stretcher to patients who need to go to hospital areas for diagnostic and therapeutic procedures. A patient escort may also assist the nursing staff in lifting patients out of and into their beds. Besides this physical contact, a patient escort socially interacts with patients. Hospitals either have a centralized patient escort service or department whereby transportation is dispatched from one central area or have a decentralized services whereby individual hospital departments are responsible for providing their own patient transportation. Also, there are computer software programs available which allow for scheduling quick and efficient patient transport in the larger or complex hospitals.

THE PATIENT REPRESENTATIVE

Patient representative programs evolved in the late 1950s with the purpose of ensuring that patients were treated with dignity. In 1971, the Association of Patient Service Representatives was founded, and, in 1972, the Society of Patient Representatives was recognized. Today, patient representative programs are common among hospitals.

The patient representative functions as a liaison between the patient, the family and the complex health care and hospital system. The representative is a listener, communicator, and facilitator. Duties of the representative include alleviating patients' anxieties, explaining hospital policies, investigating patients' complaints, and attending to patients' emotional needs. The patient representative also works closely with physicians, nurses, social workers, clergy, and risk managers in order to increase patient satisfaction and work toward a positive public image for the hospital.

NOTES

1. Telephone conversation with the American Dietetic Association, Chicago, Ill.

2. Joseph K. Own, *Modern Concepts of Hospital Administration* (Philadelphia, Pa.: W.B. Saunders Co., 1962), p. 320.

3. George P. Berry, ed., *Readings in Medical Care* (Chapel Hill, N.C.: University of North Carolina Press, 1958), p. 245.

Facilities Support Services

ENVIRONMENTAL SERVICES DEPARTMENT

Not too long ago, environmental services which were referred to as housekeeping services were the responsibility of the nursing service department. As nurses became more intensely trained, however, their professionalism became more apparent. Thus, environmental services as a separate functional area was born. The department has two principal functions: to keep the hospital clean, and to control the linen supply. Keeping a hospital clean is not an easy task. Part of the problem is that a hospital is an active place, open 24 hours a day, every day of the year. Frequently the high traffic areas need special attention; if they are not cleaned properly, they can give a negative image to the entire hospital. There is more to cleaning a hospital than simply making sure that each room and floor are cleaned properly under the right standards. Cleanliness for both hospital patients, visitors and the staff has two side effects: it creates a public relations image, and it has a psychological effect on the patients and their visitors. A clean hospital is perceived to be a well-organized and well-run hospital and secondly it can reduce the probability of infection.

Staffing

The environmental services department is a labor intensive department. It uses modern, up-to-date equipment, but the job of cleaning the patient rooms, corridors, offices, and lobbies of the hospital falls to the labor force, made up primarily of maids and porters. The administrative head of the department may be called the executive housekeeper, chief housekeeper, or director of housekeeping. The housekeeping organization is classical, in that it is based on a hierarchical principle with the chief housekeeper at the top, then one or two assistants (supervisors or forepersons), and maids and porters at the bottom.

Among the maids and porters, rank is based on a traditional division of labor derived from historical job descriptions. The maids are assigned light cleaning, dusting, and mopping of the floors. The porters usually do the heavy housekeeping and the furniture moving. By the nature of the cleaning process, there are more maids than porters. The maids are the front line of the environmental services department and generally are assigned to divisions of sections or units in the hospital. Usually, a nursing unit will have one maid assigned regularly with additional maids working the evening shift or on weekends. The maids have an impact on patients in two ways. The results of their work (that is, a clean nursing unit or patient bedroom) have both a public relations and psychological effect. The maids' approaches, professionalism, attitudes, and personalities directly affect the patients, since they come in constant daily contact with patients while cleaning their rooms. A cheerful, well-informed, polite maid can add a great deal to the total image of the hospital. Generally staff is assigned to three shifts with most staff on the day shifts.

Infectious and Hazardous Waste Removal

Whenever a patient is infectious and has to be moved into isolation, the housekeeping department must properly disinfect the patient's room and remove infectious and hazardous wastes. The department interfaces directly with the infection control committee's policies on disinfecting a given area or room, using special bacterial solutions and certain misting or other kinds of techniques that have proven effective in disinfecting accommodations. Usually infectious wastes are placed in specially marked bags and double-bagged. Incineration is the most efficient and cost-effective method to dispose of infectious wastes. Legal and acceptable waste removal varies from state to state.

The removal of hazardous wastes such as carcinogens and radioactive materials is regulated by local, state, and federal agencies. Many state laws concerning hazardous waste follow the Federal Environmental Protection Agency (EPA) regulations. The environmental services department must keep informed of changes in the regulations.

Hospitals may have on-site removal mechanisms such as incinerators or may contract with firms to provide waste removal services. The hospital as the creator of hazardous and infectious wastes is liable for safe and effective removal of these products.

Linen Control and Distribution

One of the traditional and chronic problems facing hospitals is effective linen control. Without the proper amount of linen at the right time, patient care, employee morale, and economic hospital operations are all negatively affected.

One of the tasks in dealing with linen control is the establishment of regular operating levels or par levels. A par level is a level of linen inventory required for a specific period of time in a certain area. In a nursing unit, par levels are usually planned on either a daily or weekly basis. Linen control is most adequately done through controlling par levels on the nursing unit. An adjunct to the linen control system in some hospitals is the uniform distribution system. It sometimes falls to the environmental services department to distribute uniforms for hospital personnel. In some hospitals, there are sewing rooms where employees repair linen.

Another factor in linen control, especially in guarding against pilferage, is that the hospital linen should be properly marked. Linen marking (that is, a hospital name or symbol woven or stamped onto the items) is a very effective means of reducing the temptation to people to take linens home with them. In the case of linens and sheets, decals can be affixed to the items. It is common for hospitals to use different colored linen throughout the hospital. For example, the operating room may use blue, maternity may use green, and medical-surgical nursing units may use white. It is unusual to find general hospitals that launder the patients' personal clothing.

There are two methods of distributing linen to the nursing units. Clean linen for the day should be on the nursing floor ready for use no later than the first shift (7:00 A.M.). The distribution itself is usually handled in a centralized fashion in which one or more large linen carts are regularly rotated around the nursing units from floor to floor. Another method of distributing linen, the decentralized way, is to provide each nursing unit with its own separate linen cart. With this method, a nursing unit may have a small supply of emergency linen on the floor, but the bulk of the linen is kept in the linen carts usually under lock and key.

HOSPITAL LAUNDRY

Hospitals may have their own hospital laundry, built and operated on the hospital grounds or in the hospital proper or they may contract out laundry services. A typical hospital laundry will have areas set aside for receiving and sorting soiled linen. Other functional areas of the laundry are the washing room and the clean linen processing room with its large tables for sorting, tumblers for drying, and machines for pressing the other linens. Besides the linen processing room, the laundry will have a clean linen and pack preparation room where the clean linen is put on shelves for storage or placed directly into the decentralized linen carts. Administrators and laundry managers are continually seeking improved automated equipment to save time.

The department head of the laundry is called the laundry manager. The laundry manager must possess skills in dealing with people and should understand laundry equipment and the technical aspects of laundering through proper solutions and washing formulas. The exact number of personnel required to operate a hospital laundry will vary with the number of beds in the hospital. If the laundry is responsible for retrieving soiled linens, distributing the linens, and packing certain sterile instruments, the number of personnel will increase. To operate the laundry itself, the number of personnel required for a 100- to 175-bed hospital is in the range of 12; the number for a 200- to 300-bed hospital is in the range of 15.[1] The quantity of laundry needed must be determined. One standard recommended by the government is to have six complete sets of linen for each occupied bed. According to government studies, the six sets would be used as follows: one set on the patient's bed, one set enroute to the laundry, one set being processed in the laundry, one set at the nursing unit ready to be used, and two sets in active storage for weekends or emergency use.[2]

The hospital laundry serves a large segment of the hospital. The nursing units need linen. The operating room uses a vast supply of clean linens. The delivery room and the x-ray department need gowns and drapes. The dietary department needs towels and drapes for the many medical trays it prepares. The central medical supply (central sterile supply), where so many of the hospital's sterile packs and instruments are wrapped, is a big user of linen. The environmental services department is also a principal customer of the laundry department.

MAINTENANCE DEPARTMENT

A department in the hospital that is often overlooked by patients and visitors is the maintenance department. This is especially true in a new, modern hospital. It is difficult to imagine that there would be much maintenance involved in repairing the equipment, the buildings, or the grounds in a new facility. Yet when one looks at some of the older hospitals, the role that maintenance has in keeping the hospital operating properly becomes apparent. Hospital equipment and buildings were once relatively simple. With the increased complexity of hospital facilities and equipment, the role of maintenance has become more complex and an additional burden has been placed on the maintenance function of the hospital.

Functions

The traditional or primary function of the maintenance department is to maintain the buildings and machinery of the hospital. This includes the hot water and steam plant, the plumbing, the waste disposal system, the hospital's electrical power system (including the emergency power systems), the repair of hospital furniture, and the upkeep of painting and wall coverings of the interior and exterior of the hospital. Additionally, the department is responsible for the maintenance of the grounds and for proper landscaping, including snow removal. The maintenance department plans and schedules the work to be done, too.

Preventive maintenance is maintenance work done on a regular basis to keep the hospital in sound repair and the machinery and equipment from breaking down. It includes prescheduled inspections, maintenance, minor adjustments, and standard repair. Recordkeeping is critical to an adequate preventive maintenance program; the purchase date of the item, major repairs on the equipment, and inspection reports all must be recorded.

A work order is the key document in maintenance control. It functions to plan, estimate, schedule, and control labor. Examples of items on a work order include: date requested, date needed, work order number, equipment required, materials required, estimated hours, job description, and foreman.

Some hospitals utilize computerized preventive maintenance programs as well as automated systems for processing work orders. Computerization enables the maintenance department to respond more efficiently and quickly to complaints and requests.

Contract maintenance is the use of outside maintenance experts to repair hospital equipment. Traditionally, this is done for large, complex pieces of equipment such as elevators. But as hospitals become more complex with esoteric clinical equipment, outside maintenance specialists are increasingly called in to supplement the regular maintenance staff. Usually the x-ray equipment is serviced by outside experts. The cost of these repairs should rightfully be included in the cost of hospital maintenance, even though they may show up as a direct expense in the clinical department.

Hospital renovations may also be done through the maintenance department. With the high costs of new construction, renovations have become common practice for hospitals. However, renovation can be just as expensive as new construction where there is inadequate management planning and staffing.

The maintenance department must also be concerned with energy conservation since hospitals are in operation seven days a week and use intense energy-pulling machines—such as sterilizing units in the operating room and central sterile supply and radiology units in the x-ray department.

The Presbyterian Medical Center of Philadelphia illustrates how a hospital can effectively reduce energy consumption by developing an on-site trash to steam plant whereby trash is burned to produce steam.

PLANT ENGINEERING

The plant engineering department is responsible for operating the hospital's power plant or boiler room section. The department is primarily concerned with the production and transmission of heat, power, and light.

Many hospitals generate some of the energy necessary for critical functions within the hospital, including generating steam for heating systems, hot water, and sterilizing. Also, it is common for those hospitals that have laundries to generate their own energy for this function. The engineering department, through its power plants, also may be involved in cogeneration of steam and electricity. Standby electrical systems for emergency power are also this department's responsibility. Some new power plants may have a standardized chiller or air conditioning capabilities.

The hospital boiler room is under the direction of a boiler engineer. Many states and cities have licensure laws that require boiler engineers to be examined by a board or a qualified group. In these cases, after passing qualification examinations, the boiler engineer receives an operating license. This license must be posted in the hospital's power plant as proof of the individual's qualifications. The engineering license primarily covers boiler operations, refrigeration, and the fundamentals of other activities related to power plant activities.

PARKING FACILITIES

All hospitals have some need for parking. It may fall to the maintenance department to operate and maintain the hospital's parking facilities. Convenient, safe, and adequate parking can be a big marketing plus for any hospital. Adequate parking facilities can also be helpful in recruiting medical staff and employees. For hospitals in high crime areas, a well-lighted, very secure parking facility is a must in order to retain qualified staff. The most acute need for parking occurs at the overlap time between the change of day shift (7:00 A.M. to 3:30 P.M.) and the evening shift (3:00 P.M. to 11:30 P.M.)

There are three types of parking areas: surface parking or on-ground parking, multilevel parking or above ground parking, and subterranean parking or below-ground parking. Surface parking is the least costly while subterranean parking is the most costly. The enormous growth in outpatient activity has put a tremendous strain on hospitals to provide sufficient parking spaces. The provision of adequate parking areas is especially crucial for urban hospitals which tend to be land-locked. As a result, multilevel parking garages have become popular.

SECURITY

Usually in smaller hospitals security falls under the responsibility of the maintenance department, while in larger hospitals security has its own department. It is common for a retired police officer to be in charge of the security department. Also, some hospitals may use contract services for security. An effective security program is important not only to secure the hospital's building and equipment but also to protect the welfare of patients, employees, and visitors.

FIRE SAFETY

Either the security department or maintenance department is responsible for fire safety. Since most patients are unable to rapidly evacuate from a hospital, hospital facilities have special features that can contain the spread of fire, smoke, heat, and gases. Hospitals need to have current regulations and manuals pertaining to fire safety and should implement staff training and fire drills.

CLINICAL ENGINEERING DEPARTMENT

Clinical engineering, also referred to as biomedical engineering, involves functions related to medical equipment. The medical equipment, also called clinical equipment, covers the following areas: equipment used for patient diagnosis, including equipment that measures physiological parameters, and analyzes specimens in the clinical laboratory; therapeutic treatment equipment; devices that apply radiant energy to the body; equipment for resuscitation, prosthesis, physical therapy, and surgical support; and patient-monitoring equipment.

Functions

The clinical engineering department is responsible for certain tasks which can be categorized by levels. Level I tasks entail the repair of equipment and related documentation of repair history and repair costs. Level II tasks deal with preventive maintenance. These include electric safety checks, new equipment checks, and equipment pre-use preparation. Level III tasks involve management and design and specifically deal with planning, purchasing, installation, design, hazard notification, and safety committee support.

Equipment Maintenance

A hospital must have adequate maintenance for all biomedical equipment since the functioning of this equipment has a direct bearing on patient care and safety. Under the 1976 amendments to the Federal Food, Drug, and Cosmetic Act, a hospital may, as a distributor, be held liable for all device defects, including latent uncheckable defects.[3]

There are four approaches the hospital can take to maintaining biomedical technical equipment:

1. It can establish its own in-house program.
2. It can subscribe to and rely on a single commercial vendor to provide services.
3. It can participate in a shared service arrangement with other hospitals.
4. It can use a combination of vendors, manufacturers, representatives, and dealers to provide the maintenance of the equipment.

The last approach cited is an expensive one. With so many people involved, the legal liability of the hospital is also increased. The purchasing department has an increased workload in recordkeeping under the combination approved.

Staff

The support personnel who are responsible for working on biomedical equipment are referred to as biomedical equipment specialists. There are two recognized levels of specialists: the first level is that of the operation specialist who has little formal training but perhaps a great deal of on-the-job training in the hospital. This level of specialist sets up, checks, and operates the biomedical equipment. The second level involves a more technically oriented specialist with specific biomedical equipment training. This individual is trained to construct and repair the esoteric equipment. The Association for the Advancement of Medical Instrumentation (AAMI) represents and certifies the clinical engineers and the biomedical equipment specialists.

CONTRACT MANAGEMENT

All of the facilities support services tend to lend themselves to contract management. Whether a hospital decides to use a total contract service or in-house staff depends on the following factors: quality of the service, availability of in-house personnel, knowledge and skills available, availability of in-house equipment, licensing requirements, cost effectiveness, legal issues, and need to expand services. Contract service firms do offer well-trained managers. This specialization can result in efficiency as well as cost savings for hospitals.

NOTES

1. U.S. Public Health Service, 1966, *The Hospital Laundry,* p. 7.

2. Ibid, p. 1.

3. Michael J. Shaffer, Joseph J. Carr, and Marian Gordon, "Clinical Engineering—An Enigma Health Care Facilities," *Hospital & Health Service Administration,* Summer 1979, p. 78.

Chapter 15

Administrative Support Services

Key Terms

Purchasing agent • Centralized purchasing • Group purchasing • Inventory turnover • Economic order quantity (EOQ) • ABC analysis • Centralized requisitions • Personnel • Full-time equivalents (FTEs) • Position control • Job description • Orientation program • Turnover rate • Taft Hartley Act • Public Law 93-360 • Equal Employment Opportunity Act • Civil Rights Act • Age Discrimination in Employment Act • Hospital auxiliary • Beeper system

---

MATERIALS MANAGEMENT DEPARTMENT

Materials management is the management and control of goods and supplies, services and equipment from acquisition to disposition. It involves the centralization of procurement, processing, inventory control, receiving, and distribution. Effective materials management results in the purchase of goods, services, and equipment at the lowest costs and ensures that inventories are monitored and controlled.

ORGANIZATION

Various subdepartments or sections are involved in the flow of materials as illustrated by Figure 15-1. The request to acquire supplies and equipment for a hospital department will entail interaction between the purchasing section, a vendor, the receiving department, the accounts payable department, and the inventory/distribution section.

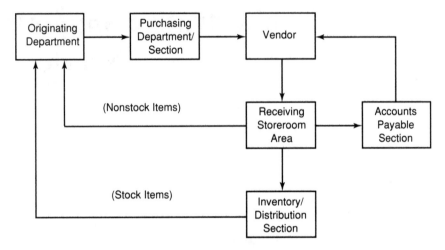

Figure 15-1 The Flow of Materials. *Source:* Adapted from *Health Care Administration: Principles and Practices* by Lawrence F. Wolper and Jesus J. Pena, p. 472, Aspen Publishers, Inc., © 1987.

PURCHASING SECTION

The hospital purchasing section or department is usually under the direction of a purchasing agent, a materials manager, or an assistant director of the hospital. The purchasing agent has to determine what, when, and how much to purchase for hospital inventories. It is the purchasing agent who seeks out sources of supplies and proper vendors. One key objective of the purchasing section is to lower the price of supplies and equipment either by direct negotiation or competitive bidding, and still acquire quality products.

To obtain suitable bids, specifications for each product must be set down, preferably in writing. One of the side benefits a hospital realizes from competitive bidding is that the purchasing agent and the department heads requesting an item have to give more thought to the item, its usage, and the standards they require for the item. One of the problems with using only price as a determinant is in the question of service. If the product needs repair, whether it be a major piece of equipment or smaller disposable item, the purchasing agent must demand that the sales and service representatives for that vendor make good with a repair call or come in to discuss the product and its characteristics with the users. Service is an element that must be weighed along with price in competitive bidding. Notwithstanding the separate elements of service and quality, however, competitive bids are definitely successful economic tools for the purchasing agent and the hospital.

CENTRALIZED PURCHASING

There tends to be a belief that the more centralized the control and the more centralized the purchasing in a hospital, the more efficient the operation and the more cost containment that can be realized by the hospital. It can result in savings by consolidating departmental needs and by reducing the number of employees involved in purchasing functions. Further, central purchasing provides the means for strengthening the purchasing organization and for establishing clear purchasing policy.

Shared Purchasing

The concept of shared purchasing power or group purchasing is not new to hospitals. Over the years, there have been experiments and cooperative arrangements. The purpose of these co-op arrangements is to reduce the cost of purchases to hospitals. Group purchasing can be as simple as two hospitals deciding to combine certain purchasing activities in order to obtain lower prices for goods or services. But one careful observer notes that there are "a host of different issues potentially arising out of shared purchasing arrangements. Any segment of shared services management that is colorably anticompetitive needs to be evaluated by antitrust standards in order to avoid costly and perhaps devastating litigation."[1] The reviewer suggested a competent legal counsel to examine any group purchasing arrangements.

Leasing

Generally, for the purchase of capital equipment, administrators have frequently been leasing equipment rather than purchasing it outright. Leasing allows administrators to purchase equipment without having the needed cash already in hand. There are two types of leases: the financial lease and the operating lease. According to one expert on the subject, "the financial lease is a noncancellable contract. . . . Usually the term is no longer than 80% of the useful life of the asset."[2] The other type of lease is the operating arrangement, "in which the lessee may cancel the contract with due notice. For example, highly technical medical equipment that may be subject to a high degree of obsolescence are acquired through this type of lease.

RECEIVING SECTION

The receiving section ensures that the correct number and type of supplies and equipment are properly received. The section is responsible for checking the condition of the items and notifying the accounting department of the receipt of the goods. The accounting department is responsible for scheduling the timing of payments to vendors. Supervising these receiving functions generally falls to the purchasing agent or personnel in the purchasing section.

INVENTORIES AND INVENTORY MANAGEMENT

Savings result when inventory levels are reduced so that both money and space can be used for other purchases. The objective is to reduce the inventory level as low as possible without running out of items. One study showed that the value of storeroom inventories varies only slightly by the size of the hospital. Inventories in smaller hospitals (average of 150 beds) and larger hospitals (average of 450 beds) are approximately $1,200 per bed.[3] Table 15-1 highlights some management tools available for effective inventory control.

Table 15-1 Inventory Management Tools

Tool	Formula	Description	Purpose
Inventory turnover	$\dfrac{\text{Annual dollar value of items}}{\text{Average inventory value}}$	Determine how fast items are moving, on average inventory turnover should be 12x/year.	Identify obsolete, slow-moving, or excess items. Assists to determine when to re-order items.
Economic order quantity (EOQ)	$\dfrac{\text{Annual usage x 2 x order cost}}{\text{Unit cost x}}$	Determine optimal audit quantities for items. Calculate the annual usage of each item in dollars, determine dollar costs of placing purchase orders, holding or carrying costs, and average inventory on hand.	Make economic goals and efficient par levels for each inventory item.
ABC analysis		Classify entire inventory into three categories based on yearly dollar usage of items (A=high dollar usage, B=middle dollar usage, C=low dollar usage).	Determine percentage of costs spent on percentage of inventory.

THE STOREROOM

The majority of the hospital's inventory is kept in the main hospital storeroom. Items may be distributed via requisitions, par-level systems, or exchange carts. Using requisitions is a traditional system whereby individual departments or nursing units determine when and how much to order. In the par-level system, personnel from the approval of management or central supply section department go to each appropriate hospital department and nursing unit, count the supplies, write up orders, obtain the supplies, and bring them back to the unit. Supplies are brought up to the standard or par level. A variation of the par-level system is to distribute supplies on a movable cart. According to a predesignated schedule, depleted carts are exchanged with full carts. This is called an exchange cart system.

HUMAN RESOURCES DEPARTMENT

There are several reasons for a hospital to have an organized human resources department, previously referred to as the personnel department: (1) management has discovered that a well-functioning human resources department can bring economies of scale to the hospital operation; (2) it is psychologically important for the employees that one department oversee the maintenance of personnel records and benefits; and (3) the human resources department is a strong guide and consultant to top management of the hospital. This is particularly true now in the age of increased employee recordkeeping responsibilities placed upon hospitals by the federal and state governments and other regulatory agencies.

Department Functions

The human resources department coordinates the processes of selecting and hiring personnel and assists departments in their recruiting and selection needs. The department's activities are generally divided into two functional areas: obtaining employees, and maintaining those employees' records and programs once they are within the hospital organization.

A Position Control Plan

The position control plan is a management tool that allows the hospital to control the number of full-time equivalent employees (FTEs) on the payroll compared to what was budgeted. A full-time equivalent is the number of hours that a full-time employee would work in a given year, 2,080 hours per year. It is the human resources department's responsibility to maintain the master employee file and the employee position control files.

Job Analysis

Before an employee can be recruited, selected, and brought into the hospital, the human resources department should observe and study the tasks and functions to be performed by the employee, the conditions under which the employee is supposed to work, the skills and training aptitude necessary for the employee, and the requisite abilities necessary to perform the job.

Job Description

Following the job analysis, a job description is drawn up. Job description specifications vary among hospitals. Generally, they include the job title, the work department, an outline of the tasks and duties to be performed, any equipment or special tools to be used, and the individual supervising the position.

Recruitment

Another objective of the human resources department is to recruit qualified employees. There are several ways that a human resources department can obtain employees. The applicant might be a "walk-in" who simply comes into the department and seeks employment. Another way—and an excellent method used by the author to fill vacant positions—is to recruit from within the hospital's current employee ranks.

Interviews

After human resources has interviewed and selected the best applicants, interviews are arranged with the appropriate department head or supervisor, and then the selection is made. The human resources department should not make the final selection, in most instances, and should act only in an advisory capacity.

Orientation Programs

An orientation has two basic purposes. First, it allows the new employee to get background information about the hospital and its functions and to see where the employee's job fits in. Second, the orientation should begin to make the employee feel a real part of the hospital family.

Hospitals use different techniques in orienting employees—general orientation lecture, a general tour of the hospital, distribution and explanation of the employee handbook, and the use of a "buddy" system are some of the approaches used.

Motivation and Job Enrichment

Once the employee is hired, the problems of retaining, motivating, and making the employee feel a part of the hospital begin.

One of the measures that hospitals use to evaluate employee morale and retention is turnover. The turnover rate is calculated by placing in the numerator the number of employees who were hired or left the payroll in a given month and by placing in the denominator the number of employees in the hospital. Turnover rates should be calculated every month.

Troubled Employees

Another responsibility of the human resources department is to work with troubled, problem, and dead-end employees. Those with substance abuse problems should receive referrals to appropriate treatment centers. This is handled through the Employee Assistance Program (EAP). The department also handles grievances concerning employee-employer relations.

Salaries, Wages, and Benefits

The human resources department has the job of developing, maintaining, and monitoring a salary and wage program. The establishment of a salary and wage program includes four main steps:

1. Analyze each job, determining skills and education required for the job.
2. Place each job in a group classification based on its relative importance to the hospital.
3. Assign a salary range to each classification.
4. Rate employees according to some system.

Also, hospitals have traditionally offered benefits other than a paycheck in order to recruit and retain personnel. Some of the common fringe benefits that may be paid totally or partially by institutions include: life insurance, group hospitalization, pension plans, and educational assistance. Some hospitals offer a "cafeteria plan" for benefits which allows employees to select their own fringe benefits.

Employee Performance Appraisal

The human resources department guides and supports department heads in rating employees. The rating scheme may involve a formal rating procedure based upon a supervisor filling out a form or completing a written report. Employee performance appraisals should reflect an employee's knowledge, skills, behavior, attitudes, and overall contribution.

HOSPITALS AND UNIONS

In 1936, the AFL-CIO initiated a campaign to organize hospitals. Their goals was to organize a significant portion of nonprofessional health care workers, including dietary, maintenance, and housekeeping personnel. In 1947, the Taft-Hartley or Labor-Management Relations Act was passed. This law excluded employees of nonprofit hospitals from the right to organize. Congress passed Public Law 93-360 on July 26, 1974, which removed the nonprofit hospital's exception from the Taft-Hartley Act. The National Labor Relations Board (NLRB) categorized four labor units within hospitals: (1) registered nurses; (2) all other professionals, including interns, residents, and physicians on the medical staff; (3) service and maintenance employees, including business office employees; and (4) technical employees, including licensed practical nurses. Not surprisingly, hospital management has, for the most part, been opposed to the concept of labor organization within the hospital. Until 1991, the key battleground had involved the size and nature of bargaining units. That battled ended in April of 1991 when the United States Supreme Court upheld the National Labor Relations Board's guidelines allowing up to eight bargaining units for hospital workers.

GOVERNMENT INVOLVEMENT AND REGULATIONS

There is significant federal legislation governing the selecting, interviewing, and hiring processes in hospitals as summarized in Table 15-2.

OCCUPATIONAL LICENSURE

Ever-increasing application of new medical and scientific technology requires that the established health professions expand their roles, and new jobs continue to be created.

One of the major issues with these new jobs is licensure, particularly with respect to the newer professions. The states have taken the lead in some licensure, e.g. nurses, but today there seems to be a need for clarification in handling the emergence of new jobs and professions.

VOLUNTEERS

The role of volunteers is to supplement the services provided by the hospital's employees. Volunteers are found operating switchboards, aiding families and friends at the reception desk, and serving as volunteer patient representatives. They may provide nursery service on a day-care basis. They aid the social service department by listening to the terminally ill; they perform puppet shows for the children in the pediatric unit. They may be transportation aides in the x-ray or physical therapy departments. Many of them assist the management of the hospital by offering skilled typing services and clerical skills.

The director of volunteers' responsibilities include recruiting, interviewing, and arranging volunteer assignments with various functional department heads in the hospital, providing their orientation, and assisting in training. The director is also

Table 15-2 Chronology of Major Federal Regulations on Employment

Law	Impact on Human Resources Department
1935 The Wagner Act	This act stated the uniform rights of workers in their efforts to organize.
1938 & Subsequently Updated Fair Labor Standards Act	Hospitals must abide by minimum wage, overtime, and child labor standards that apply to employees not specifically exempt from the act's coverage.
1947 The Taft-Hartley Act or Labor-Management Relations Act	This act amended the Wagner Act with regard to the rights of management or employers. In addition, it also clarified the rights of labor. (The employees of nonprofit hospitals were excluded from the provisions of this legislation.)
1963 Equal Pay Act	Hospitals are prohibited from paying different or lower wages to a woman who is performing the same job as a male counterpart.
1964 Civil Rights Act (Title VII)	Hospitals are prohibited from discriminating with respect to hiring, training, or other terms and conditions of employment based on race, color, religion, sex, or national origin.
1967 Age Discrimination in Employment Act	Hospitals are prohibited from discriminating against personnel 40 years of age and older with respect to compensation and other terms and conditions of employment.
1972 Equal Opportunity Act	Hospitals must be alert to discriminatory practices, including discrimination based on sex. They must scrutinize wage structures to see that whites and minority groups doing the same work are treated the same in compensation. Hospitals must notify every employment agency they deal with that they are an equal opportunity employer.
1974 Public Law 93-360	This law removed the nonprofit hospital's exception from the Taft-Hartley Act. This meant that approximately 101 million unorganized employees in not-for-profit hospitals could be organized under the umbrella of the Taft-Hartley Act.
1974 Taft-Hartley Act Amendments	The National Labor Relations Board (NLRB) categorized four labor units within hospitals: (1) registered nurses; (2) all other professionals, including interns, residents, and physicians on the medical staff; (3) service and maintenance employees, including business office employees; and (4) technical employees, including licensed practical nurses. *continued*

Table 15-2 Continued

Law	Impact on Human Resources Department
1986 Immigration Reform and Control Act	Hospitals are prohibited from discriminating with respect to recruitment or hiring based on national origin or citizenship status.
1988 Drug Free Workplace Act	Hospitals that are recipients of federal financial assistance must take specified steps to maintain a drug-free workplace, including the establishment of a drug-free awareness program.
1990 Americans with Disabilities Act	Hospitals are prohibited from discriminating against qualified individuals with disabilities with respect to application procedures, hiring, training, and other terms and conditions of employment.
1991 Eight Bargaining Units	After years of legal action and debate, the United States Supreme Court in April 1991 upheld the National Labor Relations Board's guidelines, allowing up to eight union bargaining units for hospital workers.

responsible for maintaining a strong liaison with the department heads with whom the volunteers work and relate. It is the director's job to keep the volunteers informed of pertinent hospital policies and procedures. One key issue in volunteer service is the volunteers' authority in the hospital. The authority of volunteers may be noted in the hospital's bylaws. In those cases, the bylaws would delineate the functions and purposes of the volunteer effort.

AUXILIANS

Auxilians are citizen volunteers who assist the hospital in achieving its mission and have a commitment to the community's health. They often form a group called the hospital auxiliary. The trustees or organized leadership of auxilians are legally accountable for their decisions and activities. Some auxilians function as hospital volunteers, while others may be deeply involved in fund-raising activities. They constitute a strong community relations aim for the hospital.

TELECOMMUNICATIONS MANAGEMENT

Traditionally, the beeper (personal paging) system has been the key communication system for hospitals. This was, and is, often coordinated through the hospital's telephone switchboard. However, hospitals have begun to establish more sophisticated, computer-driven systems such as satellite transmission, data communications, and computer-age telephone systems. Telecommunication systems function to assist the caregivers availability as well as offering an up-to-date business communications system. The nerve center for the telecommunication functions is the hospital switchboard. This area is manned 24 hours a day and is also a key public relations function for the hospital since it is frequently the first place a patient or family member makes contact with the hospital.

NOTES

1. Andrew K. Dolan, "What Are the Antitrust Implications of Shared Purchasing for Hospitals?" *Hospitals, JAHA,* 16 Oct. 1979, p. 76.

2. James B. Henry, "Know Your Lease," *Hospitals, JAHA,* 16 Aug. 1974, p. 64.

3. 1989-90 Third National ASHMM Survey of Hospital Materials Management conducted by The American Society for Hospital Materials Management of the American Hospital Association and Coopers & Lybrand.

Part VII

Hospital Finances

Generating Revenue

The principal difference between the economics of hospitals and that of retail businesses that we are all familiar with lies in how the hospital receives payment for its services to the patient. In the majority of cases, the hospital does not receive payment directly from the patient for services rendered but rather from a third-party payer. A third-party is any agent other than the patient who contracts to pay all or part of a patient's hospital bill.[1]

TYPES OF THIRD-PARTY PAYMENTS

Hospital and medical insurance payments have grown quite complex. There are three fundamental methods in which hospital payments are calculated, and each method has a different effect on the hospital's financial status. The different methods include: cost reimbursement, specific services/negotiated bids, and diagnostic related groups (DRGs).

Cost Reimbursement

Under cost reimbursement, hospitals are paid based on their total costs or reasonable costs. Reasonable costs are determined through a very elaborate cost-finding process called the cost report, which is prepared by the hospital at the end of its fiscal year. Costs not generally acceptable to third parties are any costs not directly related to the care of patients. Today, many third-party payers, e.g., Medicare, have substituted cost reimbursement for inpatient care with other payment methods, such as diagnostic related groups.

Specific Services/Negotiated Bids

This method of payment is based on charges for specific services, such as laboratory, pharmacy, surgery, and nursing services. Typically, hospital management sets the institution's charges. The charges may be discounted or negotiated. Negotiated bids entail an arrangement between a hospital and a third-party payer. Usually a fee arrangement is set for a specific time period, and contracts are not renegotiated if the hospital has increased costs. Therefore, it is crucial for hospitals to plan and control costs under this type of payment method. Health maintenance organizations and preferred provider arrangements fall into this category.

Diagnostic Related Groups (DRGs)

The DRG system of payment is based on prospectively determined prices or rates rather than retrospectively determined costs. This system evolved from research conducted at Yale University in which related diagnosis were grouped together as predictions of length of stay. This system became universal for Medicare in 1983 following the Tax Equity and Fiscal Responsibility Act of 1982. All patient diagnoses are grouped into hundreds of DRGs with each DRG having a fixed payment. Hospitals are paid these fixed fees regardless of the costs incurred for treating patients.

Table 16-1 highlights the major third-party payers and their predominant payment method.

THE MAJOR PAYERS

Medicare

On July 1, 1966, Public Law 89-97, the Medicare program, became effective across the nation. The Medicare program was an outgrowth of a federal legislative process to meet the growing problems of the aged and the disabled in receiving appropriate health services that they could afford. As part of the Social Security Amendments of 1965 (commonly referred to as Title XVIII), Medicare benefits were provided to senior citizens (over the age of 65) under two separate but closely related programs. These programs are referred to as Part A of Title XVIII,

Table 16-1 Third-Party Payers and Insurance Payments

Third Party	Insurance Payment Method			
	Cost Reimbursement	Negotiated Bids	Diagnostic Related Groups	Specific Services
Medicare	x	x	x	
Medicaid[1]	x		x	
Blue Cross[2]			x	
Commercial				x
Managed Care		x		

[1]States will vary, but many tend toward a DRG system.
[2]There are numerous Blue Cross plans and they will vary, but they tend to follow the DRG system or a modification of that.

which pays for hospital services as well as nursing home care and other institutional care, and Part B of Title XVIII (known as Supplementary Medical Insurance), which basically pays for physician fees and certain diagnostic services. The supplementary program, or Part B, is voluntary. After age 65, the beneficiary can subscribe to this at a nominal cost.

Since its passage in 1966, Medicare has become generally very popular with consumers. For the average patient, there are four distinct pluses in the Medicare program:

1. It provides almost universal coverage for the elderly.
2. If offers far better benefits than any private health insurance program could offer to this age group.
3. It assures senior citizens a certain level of access to quality care institutions.
4. It requires relatively small out-of-pocket expenses for the elderly to be covered by the insurance.

So much for the pluses of Medicare. What about the minuses? They can be summed up in a single phrase: excessive costs. In the sober words of a Senate committee on the financing of Medicare studies: "The Medicare and Medicaid programs are in serious financial trouble. The two programs are also adversely affecting health care costs in financing for the general population."[2]

Medicaid

Along with Medicare legislation in 1966, Medicaid legislation was enacted under the Title XIX. The primary purpose of the Medicaid legislation was to finance health care services for the poor and medically indigent. However, unlike Medicare which was universally applied to all citizens over the age of 65, it was left to each of the 50 states to determine who was "needy" or medically indigent and thus eligible for Medicaid benefits. Each state designed its own health services benefit plan. Thus, the Medicaid program is administratively handled at the state level.

Typically, the costs of the Medicaid program are shared by the federal government and the individual states on an approximately 50-50 basis. The big discrepancy in the Medicaid program occurs with outpatient and clinical services (physicians' services). Each state can design its own Medicaid outpatient and physician reimbursement schedules.

Unlike the rather universal popularity of the Medicare program, Medicaid has since its inception been beset by critics from all sides. The principal criticism has focused on the problems of costs and eligibility in the program. As noted, the definition of "medical indigence" was, at the beginning, left to the individual states. But since certain states, like California and New York, provided rather liberal income limits for participants, the federal government, in the 1967 amendments to the Social Security Act, set an upper limit at one and one-third times the states' Aid for Families of Dependent Children (AFDC) limit. Accordingly, many were eliminated from the medically indigent ranks, especially in New York State.

Additionally, as might have been predicted, Medicaid has become, in some states, a political football. Certain states, for example, New York, have established a freeze on Medicaid payments until the end of a certain number of years and have set payment ceilings to be determined by the state, in contrast to open-ended Medicare cost reimbursement formulas.

Blue Cross

Blue Cross is a nongovernmental, nonprofit corporation that offers an insurance program that covers certain hospital services and pays benefits based on a contract between an individual plan and the Blue Cross insurance program in a particular area. Blue Shield is the same arrangement for the physician component; in other words, it is very similar to the Part B portion of the Medicare legislation. Blue Cross contracts vary substantially in reimbursement, but basically, for inpatient care, they are similar to Medicare. Reimbursement to hospitals by Blue Cross plans represents a major percentage of hospital revenues in this country.

Blue Cross plans establish their premiums based on the average cost of actual or anticipated hospital care used by all their subscribers within a selected geographic area or a particular industry or company. The rate does not vary for different groups or subgroups of Blue Cross subscribers; for example, it does not vary based on claims of experience, age, sex, or health status. This method is referred to as the community-rating method. Insurance plans that do not use a community-rating method may use an experience-rated scheme.

Self-Pay and Other Private Insurance

The fourth major type of reimbursement is used by those patients who pay their own individual hospital bills or have commercial insurance companies other than Blue Cross to cover their hospitalization. Though many insurance companies cover hospital services, they, unlike Blue Cross, do not contract directly with the hospitals. Reimbursement to the hospitals is generally made either through the patient, who then pays the hospital, or by assignment, in which case the patient "assigns" the reimbursement directly to the hospital. In both cases, patients are ultimately responsible for their bills. Generally, hospitals receive payment from patients on a customary-charge basis, not on a reasonable-cost basis.

Management Care Plans

Managed care systems are reimbursement systems which started as a control mechanism on the increasing medical care costs. The country has continued to experience a rapid growth in two forms of managed care: health maintenance organizations (HMOs) and preferred provider arrangements (PPAs). These programs, like the prospective and retrospective utilization review efforts, attempt to reduce hospital use and thereby reduce costs. Some experts believe that the financial viability of America's hospitals will be greatly influenced by successful negotiation of managed care contracts.

NOTES

1. Howard Berman and Lewis Weeks, *The Financial Management of Hospitals* (Ann Arbor, Mich.: Health Administration Press, 1976), p. 62.
2. U.S. Senate Committee on Finance, Medicare and Medicaid: Problems, Issues and Alternatives, Report of the Staff to the Committee on Finance, 91st Cong., first sess., 1970, p. 1.

Hospital Budgeting

Budgeting is an essential and crucial function for hospital management due to the continuous changes in the reimbursement system, increasing costs, and the increased competition among hospitals. Budgeting is an ongoing process. The budget is a financial road map for the hospital to use every year. A budget is a plan in dollars and cents or an estimate of and control over future operations in the hospital.

TYPES OF BUDGETS

There are three kinds of budgets: operating, cash flow, and capital. The operating budget is the hospital's primary budget and is built from individual budgets for each hospital department and section. It is the result of a four-step process as follows: (1) projecting units of service, (2) allocating resources, (3) setting rates, and (4) monitoring performance. The cash budget is a prediction of expected cash receipts and disbursements based on the operating budget and the capital budget. The capital budget is a plan for making capital investment decisions and for financing capital purchases.

FINANCIAL AND STATISTICAL REPORTS

The budgeting process produces actual and projected financial and statistical statements. Individual hospitals will vary on the specific formats of these documents, but generally they include (1) a statement of revenue and expense (or profit and loss) for the period (see Table 17-1), (2) a balance sheet (see Table 17-2), and (3) a statistical report (see Table 17-3).

One common technique used to assess a hospital's financial condition (strength or weakness) is ratio analysis. This involves a focus on key financial relationships of values given within the statement of revenue and expenses (income statement) and the balance sheet. Usually historical comparisons are made as well as comparisons to industry standards. Table 17-4 explains the four major categories of financial ratios.

Statistical Report

The data on a simplified statistical report (Table 17-3) shows the hospital's overall inpatient and key outpatient volumes. Because hospitals have such a high

Table 17-1 ABC Hospital Statement of Revenue and Expense (Profit and Loss) for June

	Budget	Actual	Variance
Operating revenue			
Room and board	$540,000	$570,000	$30,000
Professional services	$600,000	$605,000	$5,000
Other operating income	$110,000	$100,000	($10,000)
Gross operating revenue	$1,250,000	$1,275,000	$25,000
Less: Allowances			
Contractual adjustments	$65,000	$70,000	($5,000)
Uncollectible (charity and bad debts)	$20,000	$25,000	($5,000)
Total allowances	$85,000	$95,000	($10,000)
Net operating revenue	$1,165,000	$1,180,000	$15,000
Operating expenses			
Operating costs	$160,000	$180,000	($20,000)
Payroll costs	$550,000	$570,000	($20,000)
Depreciation	$60,000	$60,000	—
Interest	$30,000	$30,000	—
Total operating expense	$800,000	$840,000	($40,000)
Net gain from operations	$365,000	$340,000	($25,000)
Nonoperating revenue	$10,000	$10,000	—
Excess of revenue over expenses	**$375,000**	**$350,000**	**($25,000)**

Table 17-2 ABC Hospital Operating Fund: Balance Sheet—June 30, 19XX

Assets		Liabilities	
Category	*Amount*	*Category*	*Amount*
Current assets		Current liabilities	
Cash	$400,000	Notes payable	$200,000
Accounts receivable	$2,500,000	Accounts payable	$350,000
Less: Allowance for bad		Accrued expenses	$80,000
debts	($100,000)	Third party advances	$200,000
Allowance for		Current portion long-term	
contractuals	($300,000)	debt	$760,000
Net accounts receivable	$4,150,000	Total current liabilities	$1,590,000
Due to/from other funds	$100,000	Long-term debt	
Inventory	$200,000	Mortgage payable	$5,220,000
Prepaid expenses	$30,000	Leases	$810,000
		Total long-term debt	$10,200,000
Total current assets	$4,480,000		
		Total liabilities	$6,030,000
Property, buildings, and			
equipment			
Land	$300,000		
Land improvements	$100,000		
Buildings	$10,000,000		
Fixed equipment	$500,000		
Movable equipment	$300,000		
Less: Accumulated			
depreciation	($3,000,000)		
Net property, bldg., and			
equip.	$9,100,000	Fund balance	$2,995,000
Other assets			
Board-designated assets	$1,500,000		
Deposits	$15,000		
Total other assets	$1,515,000		
Total operating fund assets	$10,615,000	Total liabilities and fund	
		balance	$10,615,000

fixed-cost component, management must be sensitive to changes in service volumes. Accordingly, it is important to use this statistical data to analyze operating costs and operating revenue. For this purpose, it is common to display the hospital per-patient day costs and revenue amounts for a given accounting period.

Table 17-3 ABC Hospital: Statistical Report for the Two Months Ended Aug. 31, 19XX

	Current Month	Prior Month
Operating statistics		
Patient days	4,100	4,000
Maximum days per licensed capacity (150 beds)	4,500	4,500
Percentage of occupancy	91	89
Average census	137	134
Average length of stay (for discharges)	7.5	7.3
Admissions	540	545
Emergency department visits	1,200	1,100
Outpatient visits	900	1,000
Per patient day		
Gross operating revenue	$256.00	$250.00
Total operating costs	$213.00	$210.00

Capital Formation

There are three primary sources for financing hospital construction and major equipment: (1) equity, using the hospital's own funds from retained profits; and (2) debt, the hospital borrows the funds, e.g., mortgage financing; and (3) receiv-

Table 17-4 Financial Ratios

Category	Purpose	Example
Liquidity Ratios	Measure the hospital's ability to meet its short-term maturing obligations	Current ratio = current assets / Current Liabilities
Capital Structure	Assess the hospital's long-term solvency or liquidity and ability to increase debt financing	Long-term debt to equity ratio = long-term debt / Fund Balance
Activity Ratios	Measure the relationship between the hospital's revenue and assets and indicate efficiency	Total Asset Turnover = Total operating revenue / Total Assets
Profitability Ratios	Indicate the hospital's level of net income	Operating margin ratio = Net operating income / Total Operating Revenue

ing contributions, including fund raising. With respect to debt financing, most hospitals usually have a lead bank from which the hospital may obtain a loan or establish a line of credit. In mortgage financing the mortgage is placed with a bank or other lending institution. A popular option for hospitals to obtain debt financing is to issue or float a bond. Not-for-profit hospitals are permitted to use tax-exempt revenue bonds on which the interest earned is exempt from federal income taxes. Most hospital bonds are given credit ratings which assess the bond's relative risk. The two primary bond-rating agencies are Moody's and Standard & Poors.

Chapter 18

Business Functions

Key Terms

Controller • Chief financial officer (CFO) • Accrual accounting • Chart of accounts • Posting entries • Accounts receivable • Collection agency • Fund accounting • Hospital information system (HIS) • "On-line" management reports • Personal computers (PCs)

INTRODUCTION

We have looked at two of the three major financial functions of the hospital. First, we have identified where and how the hospital receives its revenue. Second, we have analyzed how a hospital structures its operating, cash, and capital budgets. Now, let us review the internal hospital business functions.

The hospital's functions and responsibilities in this area include: (1) the maintenance of adequate accounting systems for all income and expenditures; (2) the development and coordination of the budget control mechanism; (3) credit and collections procedures; (4) collection of cash and banking procedures; (5) the maintenance of internal controls; (6) the compilation of pertinent departmental statistics in conjunction with the medical records department; and (7) the preparation of financial reports that can be invaluable tools for the administrator.

Organizationally, the individual responsible for these internal functions is either the controller or chief financial officer (CFO). The CFO is the individual who reports directly to the CEO. A controller's responsibilities extend to all phases of financial management of the hospital, including general accounting and bookkeeping, patient accounts, and various aspects of financial reporting. Generally, under the controller is a business office manager and possibly a patient ac-

167

counts manager, as well as a senior accountant (the individual in charge of the accounting division). The controller consults frequently with the CFO or the hospital administrator and the numerous hospital department heads. The controller's knowledge of all phases of the hospital's finances provides a basis for recommending ways to improve the hospital's services. Recently, controllers have been emphasizing means of decreasing costs and improving third-party reimbursement. Controllers are experts in analyzing data and inspecting reports. Through these accounting records, from which the financial statements are prepared, the hospital can determine its financial soundness.

THE ACCOUNTANT

Depending on their accounting records and the order in which they are kept, hospitals usually follow the uniform classification of accounts shown in the American Hospital Association's Chart of Accounts for Hospitals. The hospital accountant is the principal person assigned the responsibility for the hospital's accounting system. The accountant must be familiar with the current accounting procedures and statistical financial analyses used in the hospital field. The accountant works under the controller and also works closely with the patient accounts and billing department in the financial information system department. The senior accountant supervises the recording (posting) of entries in hospital ledgers and trial balances to ensure the accuracy of the records. Generally, the accountant completes any tax statements the hospital must submit and files cost reports with insurers.

HOSPITAL ACCOUNTING

Even though the hospital may be a nonprofit institution, it must adhere to strict accounting rules. The accounting records are, in the final analysis, the reports that express in dollars and cents the financial status of the hospital. Not all hospital accounting is uniform. However, with the passage of Medicare legislation in 1966, many hospitals now account for their activities in very similar ways. Indeed, the similarities between hospitals are much more apparent than their individual peculiarities.

Hospital accounting is commonly called "fund accounting." This kind of accounting was adopted by hospitals because they are the beneficiaries of many philanthropic efforts in the community. Since hospitals may be the recipients of endowment funds and gifts for very special purposes, it is necessary for them to have more than one fund. Establishment of these individual funds places the hospital and its board in a fiduciary position that must adhere to the strict wishes of the donor. In order to carry out this responsibility, it has been necessary to separate endowment funds and gifts from other assets of the hospital. The American Institute of Certified Public Accountants (AICPA) now requires that such restricted resources be disclosed for external reporting purposes.[1]

In fund accounting, each distinct phase of financial activity is handled as a separate accounting entry with its own particular objective. Each of the separate funds, or accounts, is self-balancing. Fund accounting is a technique that accounts for separate entities in a single hospital or institution. Each separate fund represents a distinct phase of the hospital's financial obligations and operations. The hospital is legally responsible for a separate accounting of each of these funds.

Most nonprofit hospitals have four distinct funds or basic sets of books that are interrelated. These are the general fund, the plant fund, the endowment fund, and the special fund. For the employee and the community, the operations of the hospital appear to be reflected in the general fund. This fund has several categories, including assets; liabilities; net worth; gross income, which comes from reimbursements; allowances, such as contractual adjustments; net income; other income, which frequently comes from nonoperations, such as gift shops and interest income; total income expenses, a major component of which is salaries and wages, discussed earlier; and, finally, the net gain or loss for the accounting period. In summary, the hospital's operating fund is an account for the hospital's day-to-day financial activities that are not required to be accounted for in any separate or special fund or subcategory group. It is the most active fund in the hospital.

Hospitals operate on an accrual basis of accounting. Under this system, income is recorded in the period in which it is earned, as opposed to a cash basis, under which income is recorded when cash is received. Similarly, the accrual basis provides for the recording of expenses in the period in which they are incurred and for the recording of assets in the period in which they are acquired. In a cash basis method, the recording of expenses and asset acquisitions is made at the time the cash is disbursed for each item. It is important to understand these two approaches to accounting. The accrual basis method is more accurate and more complete.

HOSPITAL INFORMATION SYSTEMS (HIS)

The age of computers in the hospital field began in the mid-1950s, and the use of computers has since increased rapidly to include most hospitals in the country. Yet, though there has been great progress toward the use of a total hospital information system (HIS) and other applications, the state of the art still tends to be most sophisticated in the financial area. For this reason, hospitals usually have separate financial information department under the guidance of the controller or CFO.

When business functions are adapted to the computer, the statistics either are recorded at the department level and then brought or electronically sent to the computer center for input, or they can be input directly into the computer system from the department. The latter is referred to as being "on line." From these statistics and patient charges, the patients' bills are generated. As a byproduct, a host of important statistical and management reports are also developed. After the patient accounting system has been put into the computer, the rest of the accounting system of the hospital (starting with the hospital's general ledger) can also be put into the computer. Other financial related activities include the hospital's payroll and the hospital's purchasing and inventory control system. The benefits of automation include: greater control over collection activities, reduced patient accounts receivable, improved cash flow, and improved customer service relations.

The trend in hospital information systems has been the replacement of mainframes (macro systems) with personal computers (PCs or micro systems). In addition to financial functions, information systems are being used increasingly in planning decisions with regard to medical records, administrative research, the laboratories, nursing activities, marketing, and patient care activities.

The Public Accounting Firm

Traditionally, hospitals have hired certified public accounting (CPA) firms to conduct an annual audit of the hospital's financial reports. The auditing firm monitors the hospital's internal controls, verifies the values of the hospital's assets, and traces accounting transactions. In essence, the firm renders a "second opinion" on the hospital's financial matters. It generates its own annual financial reports, which are referred to as the certified statements or audited financials. Most firms also issue a management letter that accompanies the financial reports. The management letter describes for the board and the administration those financial areas that require corrective action. In the era of heavy third-party reimbursement, the auditors can aid hospitals that are seeking to maximize their reimbursements.

PATIENT ACCOUNTS AND BILLING DEPARTMENT

The traditional hospital business office has essentially become a patients' accounting and billing office. It is often referred to as the patients' account and billing department. The primary functions of this department are to manage patient accounts and hospital accounting receivables and monitor patients' bills. Patient account management includes interviewing patients to gather information on credit and collection potential, e.g., employment history, insurance coverage, deductibles, and co-insurance. Insurance claims need to be submitted by the hospital on a timely basis to third-party payers. Many hospitals use automated systems for claim submission. The department is also responsible for maintaining accurate billing records, checking the amounts received against patient bills, comparing the bills to hospital rates to ensure accuracy, sending out itemized statements to patients, and showing payments received and balances due. Often the hospital cashier function, often located on the first floor near the entrance, is part of the patient accounts and billing department.

When patient accounts cannot be collected, they are usually turned over to a collection agency. Hospitals need to evaluate the cost and benefits of using a collection agency for unpaid patient accounts. Not surprisingly, patients frequently question and/or complain about their bills. A critical role for the patients' accounts and billing department is to maintain positive customer relations. The department is responsible for explaining billing procedures and forms, handling patient complaints, and resolving patients' billing problems.

NOTE

1. W. Glenn Cannon, Bernard O'Neil, Jr., and Allen Weltmann, *A Layman's Guide to Hospitals, An Introduction to Finance and Economics* (Coopers & Lybrand, 1978), p. 13.

Part VIII

Evaluating the Care

Chapter 19

Medical Records

Key Terms

Progress notes • Chart • Coding • Abstracting • Discharge abstract • Microfiche • Transcription • Delinquent medical records • Release of medical information • Privileged communications

INTRODUCTION

The hospital medical record has undergone great changes over the last two decades. These changes are due to the greater demand and use of the information contained in the medical record. The upsurge of interest in the medical record has been aided by the increase in the complexity of medical care and the renewed interest in the information carried in the medical record. There are demands from third-party payers and requirements based on federal and state legislation, that have increased the need for access to the patient's medical record. Hospitals are required to conduct utilization reviews and medical audits that use the medical record. The computer, as a tool in the health information and management system, is frequently interfaced with the patient's medical record. This has created a whole new discipline and scientific approach in handling the record. All of these factors have added to the growth and complexity of the hospital's medical records department.

PURPOSE OF THE MEDICAL RECORD

According to the American Hospital Association,

the primary purpose of the medical record is to document the course of the patient's illness and treatment (medical care) during a particular period and during any subsequent period as an inpatient or outpatient. As such, it is an important tool in medical practice. It serves as a basis for the planning and evaluation of individual patient care and for the communication between the physician and other professionals contributing to the patient's care. The record's secondary purpose may be to 1) meet the legal requirements imposed on the hospital and the physician and 2) provide clinical data of interest to research systems.[1]

The JCAHO states that the purposes of a hospital patient medical record are (1) to provide a basis for planning the patient's care, (2) to furnish evidence that the patient's medical evaluation and treatment were adequate during the hospital stay, (3) to provide a communication vehicle between the health professionals contributing to the patient's care, (4) to supply the legal documents in the interest of the patient, the hospital, and the health care practitioners, and (5) to provide a data base for continuing education and research.[2]

DEFINITION OF A MEDICAL RECORD

The Commission on Medical Malpractice (sponsored by the Department of Health, Education, and Welfare) indicated in its very extensive 1973 report that the hospital's medical records and the physician's office medical records are more than a series of physician communications to other health professionals. The commission pointed out that a medical record represents a

> complex communication between a health professional, including a written history and physical, progress notes, the nurses' notes, consultations, laboratory reports, operation summaries, discharge summaries, and the like. During the course of a particular hospitalization, the record may include a large spectrum of speculation and observation as the various members of the health team contribute thoughts and observations that lead eventually to the final diagnosis.[3]

MANUAL MEDICAL RECORDS

Traditionally, the medical record has been a collection or package of handwritten or typed notes, forms, and reports. The forms are the vehicle for the physician and health practitioners to record the patient's illness and course of recovery. This includes the patient's admission form, medical history, physical examination form, and laboratory, x-ray and special report forms. If the patient undergoes surgery, there will usually be authorization and consent forms (including a signed authorization or informed consent) obtained prior to surgery. The patient's anesthesia record will usually be attached to the surgeon's operative report, which is usually dictated and typed. Frequently, physicians' orders will follow the admission form. These orders are on forms, maintained in chronological fashion, by which the physician communicates to the nurses and other health care professionals instructions for determining the patient's diagnosis and carrying out the therapy. Usually near the physician's order sheets are progress note sheets. The progress note sheets are often the largest part of any patient's medical record. The nurses' notes or nursing records are really progress notes from a nursing standpoint. The nursing notes contain the nurses' around-the-clock observations of the patient. Finally, in the record there will be a discharge order written by the physician indicating that the patient can be discharged. Following the discharge of the patient, it is required that the physician dictate a narrative summary of the patient's stay; this is usually typed and placed into the medical record after the patient has left the hospital. Although this is the last document recorded by the physician, it is generally placed in first position when the record is finally stored so that reviewers can quickly see the course of the patient's hospital stay. All these forms and reports are contained in a folder of some nature called a chart.

ELECTRONIC MEDICAL RECORDS

Today, more and more hospitals are replacing manual medical records with electronic medical records. Automation has made it possible to capture, store, retrieve, and present clinical data. Many computers offer "on-line" systems that provide the hospital staff with direct access to computerized data bases through decentralized communication terminals. Some hospitals have personal computers (PCs) at the patients' bedsides, while others have PCs at the nurses' work station. Ideally, the computerized system for medical records should be integrated with the hospital's information system.

One of the benefits of electronic medical records is that the records are organized and legible and, therefore, likely to minimize misunderstandings as well as patient case errors. Also, healthcare professionals, especially nurses, are more productive as less time is devoted to paper work.

Likewise, computerization can enhance the operations of the medical records department, especially functions like coding, abstracting, noting chart deficiencies, and correspondence.

Automation also helps expedite the process of completing medical records and this will improve the timely submission of patient bills. In addition, by computerizing selected clinical data in the patient record, the hospital will be better able to track and detail that clinical information quickly and efficiently. One of the most important aspects to be considered when developing and implementing a computerized system is getting user acceptance early. The acceptance process should begin with the planning stage. User acceptance increases the level of comfort health care professionals feel while using a sophisticated computerized system.

The information system must also be secure. Restricted access prevents unauthorized use and makes alteration unlikely.

THE MEDICAL RECORDS DEPARTMENT

Medical records have been retained for hundreds of years. Even before pencil and paper, we can assume that some of the hieroglyphics on Egyptian tombs and temples referred to medical aspects of the deceased. A new impetus in medical records departments and medical records administration was launched early in the 1900s. In 1912, interested medical record librarians gathered at the Massachusetts General Hospital to discuss their common interests. In 1928, the Association of Record Librarians of North America was born. This later became known as the American Association of Medical Records Librarians.

The individual in charge of the medical records department is either a registered record administrator or accredited record technician who has passed the American Medical Association's exam. The department director is called the Medical Records Administrator. Part of the medical record administrator's job is to organize and manage the medical record system and to provide efficient medical record services to the hospital. Specifically, this person's duties include: (1) planning, designing, and technically evaluating patient information; (2) planning, directing, and controlling the administration of the medical record department and its services; (3) aiding the medical staff in its work on medical records; (4) developing statistical reports for management and the medical staff; and (5) analyzing technical evaluations of health records and indices.

Hospital medical records are highly visible instruments used in the evaluation of patient care. This being the case, it is very common for third parties, and especially the JCAHO, during their annual or biannual surveys to study and review carefully the patients' medical records.

One of the traditional areas that is almost always reviewed is the timely completion of the medical record. Outside reviewers can be expected to inspect the matter of delinquent medical records at any give point in time during the survey. In fact, if the delinquent record problems are serious, they could jeopardize the hospital's accreditation by the JCAHO.

Yet, though the medical record presents a wealth of data for countless third parties, quality assurance reviewers, and third-party payers, one of the most common problems in medical records still remains that of delinquent medical records. Not all physicians complete their medical records in a timely and accurate manner according to the medical staff bylaws. This tends to be a chronic problem faced by medical record administrators across the country. In the final analysis, the most potent weapon against these delinquencies is suspension of privileges of physicians until they complete their records.

ORGANIZATION OF THE DEPARTMENT

The organization and staffing of the medical record department reflect in a very straightforward manner the tasks and functions of the department. The department is staffed to handle (1) release of information, (2) admission and discharge analyses, (3) medical transcriptions, (4) coding and abstracting (generally this involves diagnostic and procedural coding), and (5) storage and retrieval.

In the area of statistics and recordkeeping, the statistical section of the medical records department provides the input to many of the computerized data services that hospitals use to generate computerized patient data profiles. The primary source of this data is the patient's discharge abstract that is submitted to certain third-party agencies. This data is summarized in computer language and sent to a computer with large memory banks. The hospitals can then receive the information in a readable and quickly retrievable fashion. Hard copy medical records are usually stored as microfiche which is an efficient, cost effective means of storage and retrieval.

The transcription section of the medical record department is an area in which medical typists transcribe the summaries and reports dictated by physicians onto paper for filing in the medical record. At one time, many hospitals employed medical transcribers; today, it is common to use outside transcription services. With these outside systems, the transcription is dictated over the telephone, typed, and then sent by messenger or mail to the hospital. This system offers the hospital the advantage of not having to deal with and manage various hospital employees. Also, the hospital is paying exactly for what it receives in typing, and the outside service relieves the hospital from the task of maintaining a bank of technical transcription equipment and a cadre of qualified typists.

THE MEDICAL RECORDS COMMITTEE

The medical staff's medical records committee is the liaison between the medical record department and the physicians in the hospital. This committee is charged with the responsibility of reviewing and evaluating the medical records function. These tasks should be performed not less than quarterly. Generally, based on random sampling and recommendations from a variety of medical sources, the committee will review certain records on a regular basis for appropriateness. However, the principal responsibility for quality of peer review rests with the medical staff's audit, utilization, review, and quality assurance committees.

The medical records committee's principal responsibility is to supervise the organization of the record. The committee must review and approve all new medical record forms. In view of the fact that the traditional record is a potpourri of medical forms, this can be, at certain hospitals, a very time-consuming task. The committee should evaluate the accuracy of certain record notations relating to management and administrative matters of the record. For example, if physicians are not writing the discharge diagnosis on the medical record at the proper time or in the proper place, the medical records committee should take directive action. It is the committee's responsibility to police the traditional and chronic problem of physicians' delinquency in completing medical records.

The medical records committee does not generally get involved in making recommendations on management issues in the medical records department. For example, filing procedures, coding of medical records, storage, microfilming potentials, and preservation of certain sections of the record are matters usually left to the medical records administrator in conjunction with the hospital management.

LEGAL REQUIREMENTS

The medical records administrator is the custodian of the medical records and must be alert to certain legal requirements with regard to the handling and release of medical information and medical records. The maintenance of medical records is governed by the Uniform Business Record Evidence Act. Accordingly, the records are retained as part of the day-to-day business of the hospital.

Rules on the release of medical information vary from state to state. Thus, the medical records administrator must understand the specific rules in the state in which the hospital is located. The medical records administrator is also expected to handle privileged communications with individuals, through the courts or various governmental agencies under established hospital policy, and to follow state and federal rules and laws. The medical records administrator is the special guardian of medical records that are in litigation (for example, malpractice suites). In that capacity, the administrator has to testify (orally or in writing) at legal hearings and sometimes actually has to go to court to indicate that the hospital medical record is the accurate document it is purported to be.

MEDICAL RECORDS AND QUALITY ASSURANCE

Besides medical records serving as a communications medium for healthcare workers and physicians, they have another primary function. Medical records provide the principal data base for performing quality assurance. This key role has made the hospital medical record an increasingly vital document for hospitals.

NOTES

1. American Hospital Association, *Hospital Medical Records—Guidelines for their Use and the Release of Medical Information* (Chicago, Ill.: 1972), p. 3.

2. Joint Commission on Accreditation of Hospitals, *Accreditation Manual for Hospitals—1980 Edition* (Chicago, Ill.: JCAH, 1979), p. 83.

3. Department of Health, Education, and Welfare, *Report of the Secretary's Commission on Medical Malpractice,* DHEW publications no. (05)73-88, 1972, p. 76.

Chapter 20

Quality Assurance

Key Terms

American College of Surgeons • Utilization Review • Committee structure of the medical staff • Credentials committee • Morbidity and mortality committee • Tissue committee • Clinical • Peer review organizations (PRO) • Structure • Process • Outcome • Darling case

---

DEFINITION

The "quality" part of quality assurance is not easy to define. To define it we must use terms like characteristic, property, and attribute—all of them as difficult to define as quality itself. One approach is to look at a few things that quality is not. In medicine, it is not the same as quantity, cost, cost efficiency, utilization of health care, or medical care. Quality is not consistent across the board; it may vary from time to time in hospitals and among physicians. Finally, quality can denote either good or bad, and bad quality is as difficult to define as good quality.

Having stated all of this, what then is quality? A traditional view of physicians is that quality of health care must depend upon the credentials of the provider. There is a belief that the physicians who are highly trained are probably better than those who are less well trained. Many believe that the real test of quality of care is: How did it turn out? To put it another way, when the physician and the medical team treated the patient, did the patient recover; and did the patient have good results? Health care providers also define quality with respect to the technical aspect of care, including the quality of the diagnostic and therapeutic aspects of their care.

Patients have different views of quality. Patients equate quality with relief of symptoms, functional improvement, empathy from practitioners, and the satisfaction of psychological and physical needs, including the comfort of the hospital stay.

Quality, according to some experts, is a function of the medical service given patients at a specific point in time by a specific doctor to a specific patient. You cannot evaluate after the fact adequately if you were not there rendering the care. The American Society of Internal Medicine and its committee on quality evaluation have defined quality as follows: "Quality medical care embodies a scientific approach to the establishment of a diagnosis and institution of appropriate therapy and management, designed to satisfy the overall needs of the patient. It should be readily available, efficiently rendered, and properly documented."[1]

The JCAHO states that quality patient care is "the degree to which patient-care services increase the probability of desired patient outcomes and reduce the probability of undesired outcomes, given the current state of knowledge."[2]

Quality assurance in hospitals is really an ongoing process. Its goals are to measure and to evaluate the professional services rendered to the patient in the hospital. Service in a proper quality assurance program is measured against a prevailing and accepted standard of professional care. The end product of quality assurance is the improvement of care; it is supposed to change the behavior of physicians and health team members and thereby improve the quality of care.

HISTORICAL REVIEW

There are records on the quality of care that go back as far as the eleventh century B.C., when Egyptian physicians were reported to be regulated by a certain law as to the nature and extent of their practice.[3] Quality assurance programs in America became common and were better understood following the early 1900s when Abraham Flexner presented his classic report on the quality of medical education in this country. In 1918, the American College of Surgeons initiated the Hospital Standardization Program to encourage uniform medical record formats and to facilitate accurate recording of the patient's medical course. In 1951, based on this effort, the JCAH (forerunner of the JCAHO) was established. In the 1950s, the JCAH attempted to implement certain basic auditing procedures, but they did not prove to be very useful. In 1966, the Medicare and Medicaid programs became effective, making it mandatory for hospitals to perform utilization review functions.

Utilization review is the process designed to monitor the need for patient admission to the hospital and for the continued stay of each inpatient. Partly as an attempt to control spiraling health care costs, Congress in 1972 passed a Social Security amendment called Public Law 92-603. This legislation mandated Professional Standards Review Organizations (PSRO). With the PSRO legislation, a nationwide network of locally based physician groups was created to review the necessity, the quality, and the appropriateness of hospital care provided under the provisions of the Social Security Act.

In 1972, the American Hospital Association (AHA) sponsored the "Quality Assurance Program for Medical Care in the Hospital" (QAP) as the principal framework for monitory quality assurance in hospitals. The QAP envisioned two working committees: a utilization review committee (UR) and a medical audit committee (MA). The utilization review committee had five separate elements: (1) the certification of admission, (2) preadmission testing, (3) length of stay (LOS) certification, (4) length of stay review, and (5) discharge planning. The medical audit phase of the program stressed the development of objective criteria and provided for detailed medical audits to be processed and measured against those criteria.

CLASSICAL TECHNIQUES

The hospital has continued to use quality control mechanisms primarily through its committee structure of the medical staff organization. These classic control mechanisms stemmed from the medical staff bylaws, rules, and regulations and drew their authority from the board of trustees.

Among the major quality control mechanisms that should be in each medical staff's bylaws is a committee structure that includes: (1) a medical records committee to review the contents, appropriateness, and timeliness of medical records, (2) a medical audit committee designed to conduct studies of clinical problems and practices, and (3) a utilization review committee responsible for monitoring length of stay and other utilization review activities.

Also, there may be a morbidity and mortality committee of the medical staff that reviews unusual deaths and watches for any pattern of deaths. The infection control committee of the medical staff handles episodes of hospital-acquired infections and other infectious outbreaks. The tissue committee is another important committee that exercises control over quality. It is charged with the responsibility of studying and examining the tissue removed from surgical procedures. It renders its reports to the executive committee of the medical staff.

The credentials committee is charged with the responsibility of interviewing and reviewing the credentials and delineation of privileges for each new medical staff candidate. Also, there may be a medicolegal or risk management committee in the hospital whose responsibility is to monitor incidents that might result in liability suits, to analyze suits, and to establish preventive actions. Many hospitals have a pharmacy and therapeutics committee for monitoring antibiotic prescribing practices, for assessing the questionable prescribing of new drugs, and for considering new drugs for the formulary.

Newer Approaches

For quality assurance (QA) to be performed properly, it must be integrated with utilization review (UR). Utilization review is a mechanism for reviewing the appropriateness, necessity, and quality of care provided during a patient's hospitalization. A review may be done prior (preadmission review) or following (retrospective review) treatment. The UR function has been largely shaped by the government and various regulatory programs. Professional (peer) review organizations (PROs) mandated with the Medicare program, replaced Professional Standards Review (PSRO) in 1986. These organizations ensure that services provided to Medicare beneficiaries are necessary and appropriate. The PROs employ nurses who perform utilization reviews on federally financed patient care in hospitals. Also, the nurse reviewer may be employed by a hospital that has been given reviewer responsibility from the PROs. The government has let PROs take the lead in performing quality assurance.

Clinical outcomes have become an important tool for hospitals to increase quality. Measuring outcomes involves examining the process, that which is done, as well as the outcome, the results of care. There is a strong focus on the patient and in understanding which treatments do and do not contribute to the care of the patient.

There have been external pressures from the federal and state governments to monitor and improve health care quality. The Health Care Financing Administration (HCFA) has begun to publish hospital mortality and morbidity rates each year. They have found a significant correlation between high mortality rates and quality problems. In Pennsylvania, the Health Care Cost Containment Council also releases information on the severity of illness and the subsequent severity of morbidity for inpatients in Pennsylvania hospitals. The reports are tools to assess if a hospital appropriately admits patients and efficiently and effectively delivers care.

DEFINING AUDIT TERMS

The medical audit is one of the principal tools used to evaluate quality care in institutions. It is therefore necessary to understand clearly certain definitions used in the medical audit process. There are three generally accepted systems used in conducting a medical audit: the structure system, the process system, and the outcome system.

The structure system is one in which the hospital and its medical staff evaluate the setting in which care is rendered and resources made available to the physician and practitioner to give the care; this system deals primarily with the adequacy of the hospital's facilities and manpower. Process audit refers to what the physician actually does to diagnose and to treat the patient; this involves the source of medical care and the patient's compliance with the physician's orders. Outcome audit concerns the actual results of the care given. For example, did the patient respond properly to treatment? What was the mortality rate for treatment? Was the patient able to perform regular daily activities? And did the patient have any psychological effects?

Because there are three kinds of structures or systems for evaluation, the hospital has the opportunity to review quality while the patient is in the hospital and also retrospectively in terms of what happened after the patient left the hospital, based on the medical records. Traditional medical audits in the hospital usually included retrospective review of the medical care process, based on the patient's medical record. More recently, the questions of outcome and patient satisfaction are also being considered.

Although the principal function of a medical audit should be to improve patient care, there are also byproducts. Deficiencies are noted and can be corrected. The audit method encourages coordination of physicians with other health team members in the planning of patient care. The documentation of patient care is improved through medical records. Additional direction is given to continuing education programs for physicians and health care personnel. The need for new equipment or facilities can be brought to the attention of the management of the hospital. Finally, a proper medical audit provides to the board of trustees written documentation of the status of the medical care as practiced in certain diagnoses in the hospital.

THE BOARD'S RESPONSIBILITY

In the 1965 landmark legal suit in the state of Illinois, *Darling v. Charleston Community Hospital*, the court ruled that a hospital and its board of trustees must assume shared responsibility for the medical care of the patients in the hospital.[4] Other court interpretations since then have confirmed the hospital's obligation to oversee the medical staff in the quality of care. The board of trustees should play a role in the hospital's structuring of quality control systems. It must make sure that the medical staff is well organized and that appropriate and effective medical audit procedures are implemented in the hospital.

AUTOMATED QUALITY ASSURANCE

The computer software industry has developed information systems to monitor the severity of inpatient illnesses. These systems are capable of collecting patient care data, computing the data against standards, and interpreting the results. Hospitals are better able to assess the patient on admission, at peak clinical severity, and at discharge with the information. Quality problems such as an inappropriate percentage of deaths at a certain level of severity can be identified. Hospitals using computerized information may then be able to better respond to demands made by regulators involving the submission severity, morbidity, and mortality reports.

THE FUTURE OF QUALITY ASSURANCE

In order to assess and improve health care quality, federal, state, and local governments, in addition to other agencies and groups, will continue to request reports and information about quality of care. This outside review of quality of care data may begin to resemble the process used by certified public accounting firms that examine hospital financial reports. Likewise, more and more outside agencies will perform assessments of "quality solvency" for hospitals.

In addition, not only will clinical outcomes be measured for federally financed inpatients, but also for all patients whether inpatients, outpatients, emergency room, clinic, nursing home, or home health patients. The future of quality assurance will include more types of patients and a refinement of data collection and reporting systems.

NOTES

1. W. Felch, "Practice Problems: The Assessment of Quality," *Internist,* December 1969, p. 20.
2. "Modern Healthcare," 16 Dec. 1988, p. 10.
3. C. Buck, "Terms and Trends in Quality Assurance," *Trustee,* September 1975, p. 32.
4. Darling v. Charleston Community Hospital, 211 N.E. 2d 253 (1965) cert. denied 383 V.S. 946 (1966).

Chapter 21

Risk Management and Malpractice

Key Terms

Loss prevention • Incident report • Risk manager • Plaintiff • Negligence
• Damages • Defensive medicine • Malpractice cases

RISK MANAGEMENT

Risk management is an early warning system for identifying potential causes of liability and for averting their occurrences. The primary function of risk management is to coordinate and implement loss prevention and corrective activities throughout the hospital. Another function is to receive, evaluate, and maintain reports on incidents and/or accidents occurring in the institution. The incident report is the primary instrument used to provide clues identifying a risk situation.

RISK MANAGEMENT AS A TEAM APPROACH

Although there is usually an individual designated as the hospital's risk manager, a team approach is essential for effective risk management. Team members include administrators, members of the governing body, physicians, the professional staff, employees, the in-house council (if there is one), a lawyer, and possibly insurance consultants.

Risk management should be integrated with the hospital's traditional quality assurance committees—utilization review, quality assurance, safety and loss control, and infections.

RISK MANAGEMENT VS. QUALITY ASSURANCE

Even though risk management and quality assurance are individual practices with independent functions, some of these functions overlap as illustrated in Figure 21-1. The shaded area represents functions in which risk is lowered as a result of quality assurance. The unshaded areas denote the difference between the two activities as separate activities.

For instance, the primary purpose of risk management is to protect the hospital's assets, whereas the fundamental reason for quality assurance is to protect patients. The primary task in risk management is to identify all risk exposures, whereas in quality assurance it is to measure care against standards. Lastly, risk management tends to be a prospective activity; quality assurance is largely a retrospective activity.

RISK MANAGEMENT AND MALPRACTICE

Risk management has proven to be a beneficial tool for hospitals in the prevention of malpractice suits. Detecting substandard practices and correcting them does prevent malpractice claims. Discussing occurrences with patients and families can further discourage litigation. Risk management also helps to ensure that physicians and health care professionals are practicing according to acceptable standards.

Overview of Malpractice

The phenomenon of malpractice that began to flourish in the early 1960s has continued to mushroom in the health care field. In one view, "medical malpractice is a failure on the part of the provider of health care to conform to accepted stan-

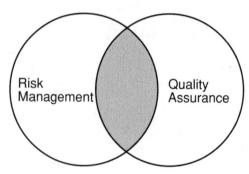

Figure 21-1 Relationship Between Risk Management and Quality Assurance

dards of skill and care or other misconduct which causes injury to a patient."[1] In 1973, medical malpractice was defined in a very complete study by the Department of Health, Education, and Welfare. In the department's *Report of the Secretary's Commission on Malpractice*, the following was stated:

> Medical malpractice has been defined as an injury to a patient caused by a health care provider's negligence; a malpractice claim is an allegation with or without foundation that an injury was caused by negligence; injury implies either physical or mental harm that occurs in the course of medical care whether or not it is caused by negligence; compensation requires proof of both an injury and a professional negligence.[2]

To win a malpractice suit, the plaintiff (the individual suing the hospital) must meet two standards. First, the plaintiff must prove that the poor or unfortunate results that occurred from the alleged malpractice were really negligence, not solely a misadventure. Second, the plaintiff must prove that, because of the unfortunate medical results, there resulted a financial loss or other damages from the negligence.

DEFENSIVE MEDICINE

As a direct result of the medical malpractice crisis, there has been an alarming increase in defensive medicine practiced by physicians. In 1973, the HEW Secretary's Commission defined defensive medicine as "the alteration of modes of medical practice, induced by the threat of liability for the principal purpose of forestalling the possibility of law suits by patients as well as providing a good legal defense in the event such law suits are instituted."[3] The costs for the additional tests performed to protect the physician are staggering.

HOSPITAL LIABILITY FOR PHYSICIANS' ACTS

It is important to recognize that in some cases a hospital may be held liable for physicians' negligent acts. The most frequent occasion for this is when the hospital permits an incompetent or unqualified physician to treat a patient. The hospital can also be held liable even when the physician is not employed by the hospital. The institution is not held liable for the negligent act that caused harm to the patient, but it is held liable for its own negligence in permitting the physician to treat the patient. It is reasoned that a physician's incompetence should be known to hospital authorities.

One of the best known legal cases supporting this principle is *Gonzales v. Nork and Mercy Hospitals of Sacramento.* Similarly, a hospital can be held liable for failure to properly supervise the clinical privileges of a physician. The court's position on this principle is clear in *Darling v. Charleston Community Memorial Hospital.* Ever since the Darling case the courts have imposed legal liabilities upon hospital boards and management for the supervision of clinical practices within an institution. In essence, the courts are saying that by appointing a physician to the medical staff, the hospital is guaranteeing that physician's competence. Accordingly, preventing malpractice claims and legal litigation is a joint effort among the hospital board, the medical staff, and hospital management.

ROLE OF THE MEDICAL RECORD

It may be two or three years after an incident occurred before a hospital administrator or physician receives a notice of suit. The next step is for the physician or the administrator to ask for the patient's medical record. The hospital medical record should depict in written fashion the course of the patient's care and treatment while in the hospital. The record provides the medium of communication among the members of the hospital health team. It is also frequently a factor in whether a plaintiff wins the case. Juries and malpractice lawyers are not likely to accept the reasoning that the chart was not written clearly enough at the time. The medical record must accurately reflect the true events of the hospitalization; there is no substitute for such documentation in winning a malpractice case.

When an administrator receives a suit against the hospital, frequently the physician is named also. It is a good procedure to make a copy of the medical record for the hospital's attorney as well as for the physician's attorney. The original medical record should be placed under lock and key in the medical record department while the case is in litigation.

NOTES

1. Charles A. Hoffman, "Dissenting Statement," *Report of the Secretary's Commission on Medical Malpractice*, DHEW publication no. (08) 73-88, 1973, p. 115.
2. U.S. Department of Health, Education, and Welfare, 1973, *Report of the Secretary's Commission on Medical Malpractice,* DHEW publication no. (08) 73-88, 1973, p. 4.
3. *Wall Street Journal,* 6 May 1975.

Chapter 22

Accreditation and Licensing

Key Terms

Joint Commission on Accreditation of Healthcare Organizations (JCAHO) • Review process • Standards • Accreditation Manual • The survey • American Osteopathic Association (AOA) • American Hospital Association (AHA)

HISTORICAL REVIEW

How do patients and community residents know whether the hospital in their community, or the hospital they are unfortunate enough to be a patient in, is a good hospital? How does a patient know who has reviewed the systems, procedures, physicians, nurses, and everything else in the hospital to make sure it is all working properly? Fortunately, there is a group whose sole purpose is to review hospitals and to tell hospitals, patients, and the community whether a hospital is satisfactory or not. This process of review is called hospital accreditation, and the group that does it is called the Joint Commission on Accreditation of Healthcare Organizations (JCAHO), formerly known as the Joint Commission on Accreditation of Hospitals (JCAH).

The JCAH traced its roots to a program called the Hospital Standardization Program that was established by the American College of Surgeons in 1918. The program was established to enable surgeons to understand and appreciate the uniform medical records format that would allow them to evaluate members who wished to apply for fellowship status in the American College of Surgeons. From this beginning, the group joined with four other groups—the American College of Physicians, the American Medical Association, the American Hospital Association, and the American College of Surgeons—to form the JCAH. On Jan. 1, 1952, the joint commission officially began its work of surveying hospitals and granting accreditation. After its first year, it was clear that it had to have a more dynamic nature, and its standards were amended slightly. Ever since that time the joint commission has done a credible job of keeping up with new standards in this country and constantly revising its approach to those standards. In the early years of the joint commission, up until 1961, the field studies were done by member organizations that were part of the JCAH. In 1961, the joint commission hired its own full-time field staff. In 1979, this staff surveyed over 2,000 hospitals.

In 1964, the joint commission began to charge a survey fee to the hospital in order to complete its field program. With the passage of Medicare legislation, Public Law 89-97, in 1965, the joint commission was given a big shot in the arm. It was written into the Medicare Act that hospitals participating under Medicare had to meet a certain level of quality of patient care as measured against a recognized norm. The JCAH was specifically referred to in the law and was asked to review hospitals for satisfactory participation. This was reaffirmed by the Social Security Administration in its standards of 1965.

While the JCAH introduced medical audit requirements in the early 1970s, it also adopted broad requirements concerning the review and evaluation of the quality and appropriateness of health care. In 1979, JCAH developed a new standard requiring hospitals to develop quality assurance programs according to the quality assessment activities required by JCAH standards. Since then, the Joint Commission has adopted this standard for all other types of health care organizations that it accredits; and JCAHO's focus has essentially become quality assurance. The change of name from the Joint Commission on Accreditation of Hospitals to Healthcare Organizations which occurred in September 1987, more accurately reflects the joint commission's mission and the constituencies it serves.

During the 1980s, JCAHO became more involved in the use of information systems. It now uses a computerized system in its survey analysis process. The joint commission also has a data base that can help explain variations in outcomes of hospital care. The data base represents a potential use of performance data to improve quality of care.

THE ACCREDITATION PROCESS

How does a hospital become accredited? For a hospital to become accredited, it must first ask the JCAHO, located in Chicago, to survey the hospital. The joint commission then sends the hospital a large, involved, detailed questionnaire that cites the standards for a hospital. After the hospital has completed the questionnaire and returned it, a survey team is assigned by JCAHO, and a date is selected for a site visit to the hospital.

The questionnaire, and thus the standards, are concerned with three major areas:

1. The services and quality of services the hospital renders to the patient. The JCAHO reviews the medical staff organization and systems, nursing procedures, the dietary procedures, the pharmacy, the laboratory department, the x-ray department, and the emergency department services. It determines whether the services provided are adequate for the patient.
2. The principles of organization and administration. Does the hospital have an effective bylaws structure? Does it have written policies and procedures? Does it require its departments to meet on a regular basis and to render written reports?
3. The physical plant and the environment in the hospital. This includes life-safety code problems, whether the hospital has adequate sprinkler systems, whether the corridors are large enough, whether there are proper safety exits, and the like.

Recently, the joint commission has been spending a great deal of time and effort on quality assurance reviews in patient care areas. The surveyors review the patient's medical records and other reports to determine whether the care given was appropriate for that specific case.

The joint commission publishes a reference manual for hospitals called the Accreditation Manual for Hospitals (AMH). This manual contains the standards used by the joint commission to evaluate hospitals.

WHAT DOES ACCREDITATION REALLY MEAN TO A HOSPITAL?

The hospital that has become accredited says to its community, its patients, and staff that it wants to meet high standards and that it has taken the effort and time to have the joint commission come in to measure it against a set standard. Accreditation says to a hospital's employees and patients that the environment is of high quality and that the personnel are qualified to provide care. Lastly, accreditation says that the hospital is a responsible institution that takes its obligations for patient care seriously and has asked an independent, objective group to come in and review it.

HOW DOES A HOSPITAL BECOME ACCREDITED?

After the hospital completes the survey and the questionnaire, a JCAHO survey team is scheduled to visit the hospital. The team consists of a physician, a nurse, and sometimes a hospital administrator. If it is a large hospital, the survey team may consist of three members and usually takes three to four days to complete the survey. If it is a small hospital, there may be two members (a physician and a nurse), and the survey may involve only a two to three day visit.

The survey is quite complete and well organized. Each member of the survey team is well organized and has a specific area to investigate and study. During the survey which is actually an inspection of the hospital, the surveyors write down in detail any deficiencies they observe in the hospital and then make certain recommendations. Before they leave the hospital, they give their list to the hospital administrator at a formal exit briefing. The survey team goes over with the administrator and key members of the administrator's staff exactly what they found that needs improvement and what they recommend. This is a very open, candid discussion on how the hospital can improve itself. The surveyors' list and reports are sent to JCAHO headquarters where they are reviewed in detail. Finally, a decision is made, based upon the survey, whether the hospital should be accredited. Approximately 85% of the hospitals receive accreditation from the JCAHO, although there are different modifiers to the accreditation, e.g., accreditation with commendation, accredited, conditionally accredited, and non-accredited.

After a hospital has been accredited by the JCAHO, it receives a certificate of accreditation indicating this achievement. If it receives a three-year accreditation, it must in the interim year before the next JCAHO visit complete a detailed questionnaire identifying what it has done about the deficiencies noted in the original questionnaire. The interim questionnaire is sent to the joint commission in Chicago where it is evaluated.

In summary, the JCAHO fills a major void in the evaluation of hospitals in this country. It is a unique organization in a world in which the government and bureaucracy seem to legislate everything. The JCAHO has been responsive to the hospitals and to the federal government through Medicare; it provides a silent service to the patient and community; it maintains high professional standards; and it acts as an advisory group to hospitals and has been influential in urging hospitals to improve their life safety measures, their quality assurance programs, and their organizations.

The JCAHO has been a success. It is unique in the health care arena and in the hospital setting because it is a voluntary operation whose goal is to make sure that the patients going into the hospital are served with the quality and dignity they deserve.

LICENSURE

The JCAHO reviews and inspections are the primary controls over the hospitals. In fact, the accreditation is somewhat like an informal license, particularly since the federal government under Titles XVIII and XIX of the Medicare legislation, Public Law 89-97, has endorsed the joint commission's survey in order to certify payment for hospitals under the Medicare legislation. There are other forms of control working in the hospital system.

Formal licensing is the most common form of regulation by the states. Generally, a license to operate a hospital is issued by a state agency, perhaps the welfare department or the health department in the state. Generally, the licensing bureau or agency retains records of a hospital's bed capacity and the capabilities of its other facilities. The health and welfare departments of the states account for three-quarters of the state agencies that have regulatory powers over hospitals. A state's licensure laws and regulations usually culminate in a licensure inspection that is similar to the inspection conducted by the JCAHO. Therein lies one of the overlaps in the regulatory system. Frequently, state inspectors and joint commission inspectors inspect the same things, sometimes within the same month or within the same short period of time. Thus the cry from hospital administrators that they are being "inspected to death" or over regulated.

The joint commission has begun to reciprocally share survey information with state and district licensure agencies regarding a hospital's accreditation surveys. In turn, these agencies report information about potential standard-related problems in accredited hospitals to the joint commission. Reciprocally sharing information enables both the joint commission and licensure agencies to identify hospitals that have performance problems and thus warrant further review.

CERTIFICATION

Another form of control used for hospitals beyond licensure is the process of certification. Hospitals have had to deal with the issue of certification since the 1965 Social Security Amendments that sponsored Titles XVIII and XIX. At that time, the government established a way for hospitals to participate in the federal insurance programs but indicated that they had to meet certain general compliance conditions in order to do so, for example, establish an around-the-clock nursing staff, certain medical supervision, and the proper use of clinical records. Essentially, certification has become associated with the joint commission's annual or biannual surveys. It should be noted that the American Osteopathic Association (AOA) certifies osteopathic hospitals through inspection reports under the Medicare program.

REGISTRATION

Registration is a weak form of control in the system. Indeed, it may not even be regarded by hospital authorities as a control. However, there is a system of registration that identifies hospitals and other health care institutions so that the third parties, consumers, and federal agencies can review the rosters of such institutions. The most common registration in the hospital system is conducted by the American Hospital Association (AHA). The AHA maintains an extensive system of data collection in the form of hospital profiles. It is also involved in registering hospitals in planning areas; for example, new construction, proposed mergers, or the sharing of services are all reviewed by the AHA. The AHA publishes an annual hospital statistics report that includes data from much of its registration activities.

Part IX

Continuing to Grow

Hospital Marketing

INTRODUCTION

The idea of a hospital involved in marketing may seem at first glance to be crass and inappropriate. In the past, marketing has been associated with businesses and retail activities, certainly not with hospital service. It could in fact be argued that hospital care is something everybody needs and therefore should not have to be marketed or sold at all. On the other hand, the case could be made that hospital care has already been oversold to Americans and that what is truly needed is more health maintenance and more attention to personal habits, life styles, and environmental factors.

Hospitals, like the rest of the health care field, have avoided traditional marketing and marketing efforts in years gone by. They have looked askance at advertising and competitive pricing, though they have been willing to make some attempts in improving their public and community relations. Yet, by avoiding direct association with the marketing process, a hospital may well fall into the trap of being unresponsive to its market—its patients and potential patients.

Marketing suggests that hospitals should try to determine its community's needs, and that it should attempt to meet these needs by developing appropriate programs. A close look at the situation indicates that in that sense some hospitals really do market in some areas, though they may not call it that. Perhaps the best example is in the area of physician recruiting. Many hospitals avidly recruit physicians to join their medical staffs. The hospital is willing to give to the recruited physicians certain benefits, for example, the right to practice in the hospital or medical office building, special parking spaces, and the like.

Thus, in the critical matter of physician recruiting and maintaining an active, and loyal hospital medical staff, a classic marketing function is at work. In the physician recruiting process, there is a voluntary exchange of values (benefits) between two parties, the hospital and the physicians. The hospital needs what the physician has, namely, the licensed ability to admit and to manage the care of the patient.

From the other side, the physician needs what the hospital has, namely admitting privileges, up-to-date equipment, and well trained ancillary and support staff. In the recruiting process, both parties have exchanged things; in so doing, they have also become a part of the marketing process. This is an example of the exchange relationship or mechanism. Recently, more hospitals have deliberately become involved in traditional marketing activities. This is the result of a changing health care environment, characterized by heightened competition and a more businesslike orientation. Other factors—soaring health costs, increased participation among patients in meeting their health care needs and selecting their providers, and higher expectations from health care consumers—have driven hospitals to increase their marketing efforts.

WHAT IS MARKETING?

To paraphrase William J. Stanton, professor of marketing at the University of Colorado, marketing is a total system of interacting management activities that are designed to place, price, promote, and distribute need- and want-satisfying services to a hospital's present and potential patients. According to another definition, "managing or planning simple exchange relationships" is the essence of marketing.[2] In this exchange definition of marketing, the behavior can be viewed as a simple exchange of resources, that is, a certain individual gives another individual something in order to receive in exchange a privilege, a good, or a service. Note how this definition relates closely to the physician recruiting example used earlier. Exhibit 23-1 highlights some of the duties and functions of health care marketing, including the four most active marketing areas of today's hospital industry—public relations, advertising, sales, and market research.

Public   Relations

Public relations has been defined by Webster as "the art or science of develop-

Exhibit 23-1 Duties and Functions of Health Care Marketing

Market Planning	Corporate Advertising/Image Building
Market Research	Sales Training
New Product/Services Planning	Sales
Sales Function	Pricing
Public Relations	Sales Research
Product/Services Advertising	

ing reciprocal understanding and goodwill between a person, firm, or institution and the public.[3] Another definition of public relations is "the activities of an organization in building and maintaining sound relations with specific publics such as customer, employer, etc., and with the public at large so as to adapt to its environment and interpret itself to society."[4]

For many years, hospitals have understood the need to develop and retain positive relationships with their patients, their potential donors, and their community at large. Public relations can improve a hospital's image, generate the public's interest, and aid in fund-raising efforts. Most hospitals are likely to have some sort of formal or informal public relations program. Many hospitals have a full-time public relations staff. The main objective of this staff is to arrange for the hospital to receive favorable publicity in the community. The staff can do different things to accomplish this. They might invite a local newspaper editor to tour the hospital, thereby improving the chances of favorable publicity. Or they could develop strong contacts with a local television and radio station. This would improve relationships with the media.

The Need for Public Relations

Most large hospitals have either formal public relations activities or a public relations (PR) department. The public relations department is a staff or advisory department. Generally, there is a public relations director in charge of the department. The PR department works closely with all other departments in the hospital, but the public relations function is clearly the responsibility of the hospital management. The technical aspects of public relations, such as developing brochures or writing press releases, is usually left to a technical expert. A public relations program need not necessarily be costly or elaborate, but it must be well thought out and systematically developed with management input if it is to be effective and get the message across in a proper manner.

A community hospital has two constituents. The first is an internal public—the hospital's board of trustees, its employees, its medical staff members, its volunteers, its patients and friends of the hospital. This internal public is relatively easy to target and penetrate with the hospital's positive public image. This is usually accomplished through a series of traditional publications, such as hospital newsletters.

The most difficult segment to reach is the hospital's external public. This consists of potential patients of the hospital, the hospital's community, and the potential fund-raising contributors of the hospital. This public or external market, is not as clearly defined and is a much more difficult challenge for public relations directors and hospital management.

Publications

Most hospitals are involved in publishing public relations material and literature for their constituents. Hospitals commonly publish booklets containing patient or employee information. Frequently, they publish their own internal newspapers, institutional brochures, or even annual reports for the internal group. Most of these publications are initiated by the hospital administrator and management team. The hospital's patient audience has the greatest need for this type of published material and information, but, unfortunately for the hospital, the hospital has only a brief period in which to get its message across to its patients.

Although some hospitals are now using videos to replace traditional internal publications, these written publications still dominate and may include the following:

- A patient's information booklet. This booklet contains information that familiarizes the patient with the hospital's environment, gives the do's and don't's of being a patient, and focuses on visitor information.

- An employee information handbook. This gives the employee the rules of employment, lists the employee's rights and obligations, and frequently outlines in some detail the fringe benefits available as an employee.

- A hospital newsletter. Typically this is done by a local printer and is not generally of the quality of the mass media that most of us are familiar with. The newsletter may be published infrequently, perhaps once a month or once a quarter. The reporting staff is usually made up of amateur writers and reporters from within the hospital. However, it is a source of information, and, if done properly, employee groups enjoy reading it.

- An institutional brochure. This is available to internal groups, the board of trustees, and volunteers. It usually presents the history of the hospital, the philosophy of the institution, and other interesting facets of the hospital's operation.

- The annual report. When a hospital publishes a formal annual report, it is usually done with quality printing and a high degree of expertise in its layout.

The report is used for internal purposes of the medical staff, board of trust-ees, and employees and is frequently sent to other hospitals and to some ele-ments of the external public. Annual reports summarize the operational high-lights of the year and usually list the key management team and medical staff.

Perhaps the most common relationship with the hospital's outside public is through the mass media or press relations. The media provide a means of getting the hospital's message to the community. The hospital has specific objectives it wants to accomplish—mainly to keep its outside public informed, to improve or build a positive image for the hospital in the community, and to attempt to gain some influence on what the mass media report in the health care arena. Press re-leases are commonly used by the public relations department to keep in touch with the mass media and accordingly the public.

When a hospital embarks upon a capital fundraising campaign or annual fundraising effort, it must solicit its public, usually in written form. Though hospi-tals may not consider this a function of public relations, it clearly is, since many letters of solicitation are sent out. Often, costly folders or brochures are developed and sent out, usually through direct mail to gain a specific reaction, namely, to raise funds from the hospital's external public.

Hospital Advertising

Advertising has been defined in different ways by different people. The Ameri-can Marketing Association has described it as "mass, paid communications whose purpose is to impart information, develop attitudes, and induce favorable action for the advertiser.[5] Hospitals are getting involved in advertising more and more. Today over half of hospitals' marketing budgets are spent on advertising. Unfor-tunately, advertising still arouses considerable controversy in the hospital field. It conjures up unethical or even illegal practices. Much of this is mythical. In fact, advertising has a major role to play in the entire marketing process, in both not-for-profit and profitmaking activities in this country. According to the American Hospital Association, hospital advertising is legitimate when it includes facts re-lated to hospital services and to space facilities. The American Hospital Association's position is that it is ethical for a hospital to make its public aware of any unused services.

Hospitals are finding that they can have advertising tailored to their profes-sional needs and can select very specific target markets. For example, they can target their advertising efforts toward physicians who may be interested in using the hospital. Frequently, hospitals think about advertising as a way to improve activity in a less-used service of the hospital. For example, prospective obstetrical patients may be attracted by a family-centered maternity room that has been advertised in the local newspaper or even on television.

Functions

In general, hospital advertising (1) informs the public, (2) persuades the public, and (3) reminds the public. Mass production has created an economy of abundance. In this context, hospitals are competitive institutions. The federal government reports that there are too many hospital beds in this country. In this situation it is logical to conclude that hospitals will turn to what our for-profit retailing cousins have learned, namely, that people can be persuaded to use one service over another. People can select those services that they want to receive. The hospital can make its product or service known and tell about its benefits and features. Then it can use advertising to remind the public who have used that service to continue to use the service. It can remind them of the reasons they were satisfied with the hospital and what brought them there in the first place.

What are some of the reasons for hospitals to advertise? First of all, the hospital's patients may need information on how to prevent disease and illness, for example, guidance on good nutrition or on how a woman can administer breast examinations herself. A second reason is that hospital patients need to understand the health care system and how preventive medicine and preventive programs interact with health care professionals, for example, where cancer screening may be available and why and where children can receive immunizations. Hospitals are becoming more involved in such programs. A third reason is that hospital patients need to be informed on how to use properly all of the elements in the health care system. Hospital advertising can deliver this type of information and in so doing improve the image not only of the hospital from which the advertising is sent but the entire hospital industry's image as well. Hospitals are likely to be interested in advertising along these lines, since such efforts are very closely related to their mission of health education.

SALES

As hospitals become more businesslike and competitive, the sales function is growing in popularity. Some hospitals now have a dedicated sales force who report directly to the marketing executives or others in top management. Sales have proven to be effective, especially with respect to certain restrictive services/products like occupational health and behavioral medicine services. Also, hospitals are experimenting with telemarketing as a sales tool.

MARKET RESEARCH

Market research is one of the duties or functions of marketing that hospitals would be wise to use more. The value of market research is that it provides information pertaining to the wants and needs of a hospital's patients, physicians, and potential patients. Most specifically, it can generate information concerning perceptions, preferences, and potential demand. There are various market research techniques that hospitals use. These include demographic analysis, direct mail and telephone surveys, personal interviews, and focus groups.

MARKETING CONCEPTS

Hospitals must become familiar with certain key concepts in the marketing process if they are to be successful in their marketing efforts. Perhaps the best place to begin is with the marketing audit. A marketing audit is simply a systematic, objective, critical way of appraising how the hospital is relating to its markets at any given point in time. The purpose of the marketing program can be developed. There are three simple steps in the marketing audit:

1. The hospital must identify the kinds of information it wishes to gather in order to evaluate its market or patient relations.
2. It must set about collecting this data and information.
3. It then must evaluate the data and information it has collected.

A common marketing audit employed by hospitals is the physician audit. After a marketing audit has been completed, it may become clear to the hospital that it has more than one kind of audience or public.

The various audiences that the hospital works with are called segments or market segments. A market segment is a distinct group of patients or potential patients that can be separated from another group. For example, it is very common to divide patients by type of insurance—Medicare, Medicaid, or Blue Cross. It is also common to divide patients by age. Frequently, patients are divided by income level or by geographic location. The different ways of categorizing the hospital's patients identify particular market segments.

After completing an audit and identifying a hospital's different segments, it is important for the hospital to realize that it has an image among the patients and also among its competing hospitals. Where the hospital fits into this image spectrum is called the hospital's position. The concept of positioning is important to understand when trying to determine what programs the hospital should invest in and sponsor. To use an illustration from the business arena, the Avis position was not clear until the company finally adopted the slogan that they were number two. This move had great success precisely, because Avis did not position itself directly opposite its number one competitor but in fact differentiated itself from its competition. Put into hospital language, if a neighboring hospital has a superior cardiology unit, perhaps the first hospital should do something in outpatient pediatrics. It would thereby position itself as different from a competitor in which it could be successful and strong.

With this concept of a marketing audit, segment, and positioning in mind, the marketing program can proceed with the classic four Ps of marketing. The objective is to put the right *product* (in the hospital's case service) into the right *place* (proper location) at the right *price* with the proper *promotion*.

With regard to the right product, it should be remembered that hospitals do not really sell services; rather they sell the benefits of satisfaction the patients get from receiving services. This is the hospital's product. Ideally, a hospital should conduct inventories or marketing audits frequently to determine what its product and benefits should be. Hospitals should regularly analyze their service programs.

With regard to the marketing place, the best example in the hospital field can be seen in satellite outpatient clinics or in medical office buildings that are placed near a hospital. Such hospitals have placed their services in the right location. They are convenient to the market.

With respect to price, because of how the federal government and other large insurers reimburse the hospitals for care, price has become less important to the hospital industry than to retail businesses. There is still, however, a psychology of price and a small segment that does buy retail. For example, the market is somewhat sensitive to price for an hour in the operating room, for a four-days stay in the nursery, or for a standard charge for a urinalysis. Thus price still must be considered in the total marketing program especially in negotiating with HMOs.

The last "P," promotion, refers to the classic public relations activities that hospitals have undertaken. It also refers to advertising and to innovative ways of promoting products (for example, premiums and incentives that could be offered to certain people). Hospitals need administrators, trustees, and public relations staff members who are sensitive to the ethical issue of promotion of health services.

It is important for hospitals to understand in detail the strategies and tactics of the marketing process. If they want to attract new physicians, to develop effective programs, to retain qualified personnel, and to stay up-to-date in their delivery services, marketing can be a great asset.

FUNDRAISING

Most not-for-profit hospitals rely on donations and fundraising efforts as a source of needed funds. Indeed Benjamin Franklin spearheaded fundraising efforts to start the Pennsylvania Hospital. Hospital fundraising can be divided into two general categories: (1) annual giving programs and (2) capital or special purpose campaigns. A hospital's regular annual giving programs are usually conducted by the hospital's development office staff. Hospitals often have a section or part of their organization devoted to fundraising. This section or department is referred to as the Development Office. Hospitals frequently use outside consultants to assist them on special or capital campaigns. Many of the tactics used to solicit funds draw on proven marketing methods including direct mail, telemarketing, direct contacts, cultivation of individuals, and special events. Major sources targeted for giving include wealthy individuals, large business corporations, and foundations.

NOTES

1. William Stanton, *Fundamentals of Marketing* (New York, N.Y.: McGraw-Hill Book Company, 1975), p. 5.
2. Tim Garton, "Marketing Health Care: Its Untapped Potential," *Hospital Progress,* February 1973, p. 46.
3. *Webster's New Collegiate Dictionary,* 7th ed., s.v. "public relations."
4. "Marketing Insights," 7 April 1969.
6. Harvey R. Cook, *Selecting Advertising Media, A Guide for Small Business* (Washington, D.C.: U.S. Government Printing Office, 1969), p. 1.

Chapter 24

Planning

Key Terms

External environment • Strategic planning • SWOT analysis • Mission statement • Goals and objectives • Long-range plan • Facility planning • Government involvement

INTRODUCTION

To quote Yogi Bera, "If you don't know where you are going, you could end up somewhere else." Therefore, the concept of planning is basic to the management of the hospital. Planning makes management sense, and common sense as well, particularly now when third parties and regulatory agencies are all pushing the hospital into more competition and formal planning. Hospitals are in the midst of a rapidly changing environment. Hospital managers look around and see the demands of the population are changing. The need for physicians is increasing. The matter of solvency and appropriate reimbursement mandates budgetary planning. Add to this the fact that hospitals are becoming more and more competitive. In this situation, the hospital's survival is truly contingent upon its ability to make the right informed strategic decisions for its future course of action.

THE EVOLUTION OF PLANNING

One of the earliest planning efforts at the community level was the Hospital Council of Greater New York, which was established in 1938 to meet the needs for community agencies to plan and to coordinate hospital facilities and services in New York City. In 1948, a planning agency was initiated in Philadelphia, but it was discontinued in 1952. The record shows that in 1954 at least ten hospital councils, located mostly in large urban cities, had made some progress on capital planning in their respective regions. After 1955, more and more agencies were specifically structured to aid in community planning, and definite planning programs were set up for metropolitan hospital areas. For example, in 1957, the Detroit Area Hospital Council and the Kansas City Area Hospital Council Association established planning programs.

The issue of planning attempts during the 1950s was accurately summarized by Leroy E. Burney, Surgeon General of the U.S. Public Health Service, when he said: "Of one thing I am reasonably certain, no one organization or type of institution in this country today has the breadth of experience or has shown the initiative required for developing the whole range of health facilities and services the American people should have."[1]

Planning continued to evolve through the 1950s and 1960s. Planning was generally synonymous with developing new facilities in a rapidly expanding health care market. There was a major concentration on the development, construction, and design of a hospital's physical plant. The focus in the 1970s was characterized by continued emphasis on hospital planning and the development of new or expansion of existing programs, services, and products. In the 1980s, planning moved beyond the institution to the external environment with an emphasis in developing outside relationships. Today, partly because of the oversupply of beds in many areas and the tightening of government regulations, planning may mean a great deal more than expansion and growth. Today, planning is used to ensure that a hospital's services are necessary and appropriate and that those services will thrive in the future. Recently it has become common for hospitals to develop associations, shared services, or linkages with other health providers as part of their planning process.

Hospitals are looking seriously at horizontal growth in the industry. For example, they are exploring home care, primary care, long-term care, and other forms of subacute care that relate directly to the hospital. Many hospitals are joining together in not-for-profit multisystems of one type or another.

THE HOSPITAL'S LONG-RANGE PLAN

Although the government and planning agencies essentially force the hospital to do strategic planning, it is actually to the advantage of a hospital to do sound, practical planning for the future—particularly now when there are so many forces (competitors to the hospital and other health agencies) impacting on a hospital's environment that must be considered by the board of trustees and hospital management. The changing patterns of medical practice include the shift from acute inpatients to ambulatory medicine, the mushrooming of biomedical technology with its impact on the hospital's operation costs and future, and shifts in demography and community needs. These changing patterns are especially important in urban areas where age, insurance coverage, and mobility are constant factors in hospital planning. Finally, changing economic conditions—particularly in the availability of money to carry out the hospital's plans—and increased legislation and regulations will impact the hospital. All of these factors must be placed into the planning mixture in order to come up with a menu that will serve the hospital in the future.

WHO SHOULD DO THE HOSPITAL'S PLANNING?

The hospital's planning effort is usually led or initiated by the CEO but generally involves active participation from the board and the medical staff. The CEO may also receive assistance from the hospital's own planning department, if they have one, or from outside consultants.

As the person who is primarily responsible for carrying out the board's decisions, the administrator or CEO participates actively in the planning deliberations. Usually, the CEO determines the planning process that will be followed and suggests various options available to the board in making long-range planning decisions.

The medical staff's role is also critical. The medical staff must identify changes in the health care needs of the community and suggest new options on how the hospital might meet these changing medical needs. Medical staff members are spokespersons for the advancing medical technology and can advise the board's planning committee on how this technology will impact the hospital's plan. Another byproduct of having the medical staff participate in planning is that staff members can become acquainted with the problems facing the hospital management in planning for the future, usually in an environment of limited resources.

The Planning Process

Hospitals generally follow a logical planning sequence. First, both the internal and external environment of the hospital needs to be assessed. This evaluation step is commonly referred to as a SWOT analysis whereby the institution's strengths, weaknesses, opportunities, and threats are evaluated.

Once the hospital's environment has been analyzed, the hospital decides what it wants to do and be in a broad sense. This decision involves reviewing, and possibly changing, the hospital's mission statement. The mission statement is essentially a vision defining what the hospital is and what it desires to be. It expresses the hospital's philosophy and details what community services, research and/or education commitments, and major services the hospital provides. In addition to defining what the hospital is, the mission statement also places limits on the hospital's activities. Furthermore, the mission statement functions as the overall guiding principle for planning.

Next, the hospital develops goals and objectives for accomplishing its mission. Alternatives for accomplishing goals are evaluated. Both goals and the strategies and tactics for achieving those goals are made part of the plan. After the plan is approved and implemented, it must be evaluated and refined on a regular basis.

CONTENTS OF A LONG-RANGE PLAN

Hospitals will vary in how they write their plans and in what will be included. However, elements that should be included in any long-range plan are presented in Figure 24-1.

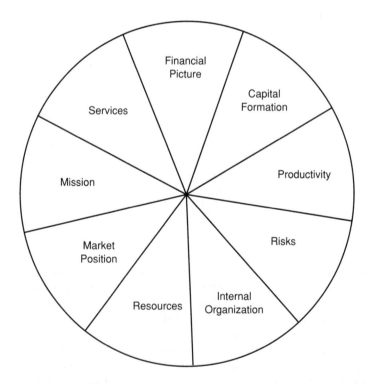

Figure 24-1 Anatomy of a Hospital's Long-Range Plan. *Source:* Reprinted from *Building a Winning Medical Staff* by I. Donald Snook, Jr., p. 10, with permission of American Hospital Publishing, Inc., © 1984.

Levels of Long-Range Planning

A hospital's plan may well have different levels of involvement and detail as shown in Figure 24-2.

BENEFITS FROM PLANNING

Clearly, proper long-range planning will improve the hospital's overall ability to deal with the future. Specifically, it will show benefits in these areas:

- It will establish a systematic basis for relating to the allocation of specific and frequently limited resources in the hospital's future.
- It will ensure that the hospital continues to look at its admission statement and its resources to carry out its mission.
- It will continue to test the viability of the hospital by integrating budgets with long-range strategic plans.

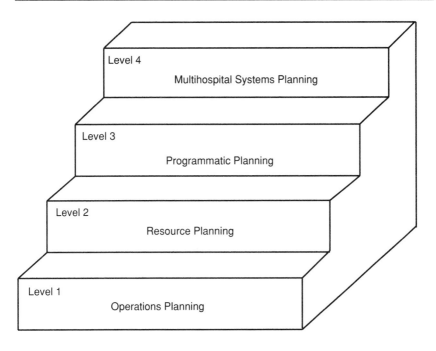

Figure 24-2 Levels of Planning. *Source:* Reprinted from *Building a Winning Medical Staff*, by I. Donald Snook, Jr., p. 11, with permission of American Hospital Publishing, Inc., © 1984.

- It will give management more control because it will have a better idea of where it is going; this will also guide management's day-to-day operations.
- It will give the hospital a standard for management against which performance can then be evaluated and measured.

PLANNING NEW FACILITIES

Facility planning involves defining the hospital's facility needs over the next several years. The facilities should not drive the plan, but rather "form should follow function." A master site and facilities plan needs to be agreed upon and followed if the hospital's planning is going to be efficient; it may include the items illustrated in Exhibit 24-1.

GOVERNMENT INVOLVEMENT IN PLANNING

A brief chronology of government involvement in health planning is provided in Exhibit 24-2.

Exhibit 24-1 Sample Facilities Plan

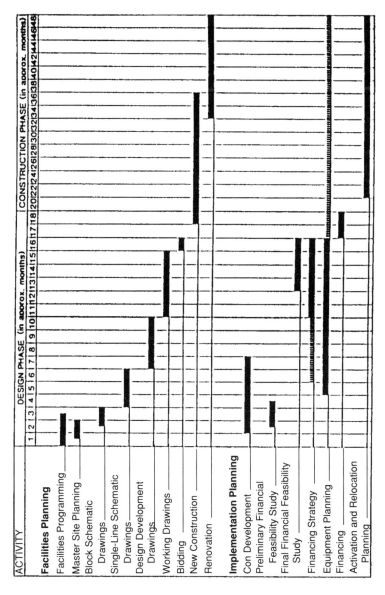

Source: Reprinted from *Health Care Administration: Principles and Practice* by Lawrence F. Wolper and Jesus J. Pena, p. 22, Aspen Publishers, Inc., © 1987.

Exhibit 24-2 Chronology of Major Federal Health Legislation Related to Planning

1946   *The Hospital Survey and Construction Act (Hill-Burton)* provided, among other things, for the creation of a state hospital planning council to assess the need for new hospital construction and to develop a plan indicating priorities to meet these needs.

1961   *The Community Health Services and Facilities Act*, among other things, provided grants for voluntary health facility planning agencies at the local level.

1964   *The Hospital and Medical Facilities Amendments (Hill-Harris Act, P.L. 88-443)* provided funds for modernization or replacement of health care facilities, as well as additional funds for facility planning purposes. In addition, the law provided matching funds for the purpose of establishing health facility planning agencies in areas where there had been none before.

1966   *The Comprehensive Health Planning and Public Health Service Amendments (P.L. 89-749)* provided health revenue sharing funds for state governments, plus grants for comprehensive health planning at the state and local levels.

1972   *The Social Security Amendments of 1972 (P.L. 93-603)* added, among other things, Sections 234 and 1122 to the Social Security Act. Section 234 required institutional planning by hospitals, extended care facilities, and home health agencies as a condition for participating in Medicare.

1975   *The National Health Planning and Resources Development Act of 1974 (P.L. 93-641)* amended the Public Health Service Act by adding Titles XV and XVI. Title XV revises existing health planning programs at the state and area-wide levels and encourages the Secretary of HEW to work on the development of national health policy. Title XVI revises the Hill-Burton program for the construction and modernization of health care facilities by linking the award for grants and loans to the mechanisms created by Title XV.

1979   *Health Planning and Resources Development Amendments of 1979 (P.L. 96-79).* This was an extensive package of all aspects of health planning, including certificate of need (CON), health systems plans, and Health Systems Agency (HSA) governing bodies.

1980   *The Omnibus Reconciliation Act of 1980* directed that a new system for health care reimbursement be developed.

1982   *The 1982 Tax Equity and Fiscal Responsibility Act* set limits on allowable increases in Medicaid and Medicare expenditures and provided for the development of a prospective payment system for Medicare payments to hospitals.

1983   *The Social Security Amendments Acts (P.L. 98-21)* of 1983 included the establishment of a prospective payment system that would pay hospitals a set price per discharge based on the diagnosis related group (DRG) into which a Medicare patient falls. These changes have subsequently become the basis for virtually all reimbursement. They have permanently altered the nature of health care delivery in the U.S.

1985   *The Medicare and Medicaid Budget Reconciliation Amendments of 1985.* Changes to Medicare continued in the mid-80s with the historic budget balancing legislation en-

continued

acted by Congress in 1985. Medicare was subject to cuts of up to 1% in fiscal 1986 and 2% in the following four fiscal years to meet deficit targets established by the legislation.

1986   *The Health Care Quality Improvement Act (P.L. 99-660)* was an important development affecting the way hospitals interact with their medical staffs. This law protected hospitals from lawsuits filed by physicians as a result of peer review activities. The National Practitioner Data Bank was authorized by this Act. It requires that hospitals report when they take away or limit a physician's clinical privileges and tracks malpractice payments and licensing actions.

1987   *The Nursing Home Quality Reform Act,* as part of the Omnibus Budget Reconciliation Act of 1987 (OBRA 87), provided more adequately regulated nursing homes throughout the country. The laws require substantial upgrading in nursing home quality and enforcement in several areas including discrimination against Medicaid recipients, licensed nurse coverage, and federal standards for nursing home administrators.

1988   *The Medicare Catastrophic Illness Insurance Act* was a landmark law authorizing the largest expansion of the federal health program for the elderly since 1985. The program was designed to ease the burden of catastrophic health care costs for Medicare's elderly and was viewed as a financial safety net for Medicare beneficiaries with serious illnesses.

1989   *The Medicare Catastrophic Illness Insurance Act* was repealed in November 1989.

Part X

The Health Care System

The Medical Care System

INTRODUCTION

Webster defines a system as a "set or arrangement of things so related or connected as to form a unity or organic whole; a set of principles, etc., arranged in a regular orderly form as to show a logical plan linking the various parts."[1] More specifically, a health or medical system, sometimes incorrectly referred to as a health care system, is a set of mechanisms through which human resources, facilities, and medical technology are organized by means of administrative structures. The system offers integrated services in sufficient quantity and quality to meet the community's demand at a cost compatible with the community's financial resources. In referring to the system's structure, its critics have called it a non-system. This observation reflects a pluralism within the hospital structure rather than a lack of system. The American system has not been the product of a grand central design but rather has evolved over the past 250 years.

The American medical system offers three classes of care: middle-class care; second-class care; and the narrow and limited "princely" care given to the elite and super-wealthy. Because our society has much more knowledge than know-how, there has been prodigious progress in medical science but a failure to make it accessible in equal proportions to all segments of our society.

The type of medical care a person receives depends upon where the person lives and how much money the person has. Better care is given to those living near university medical centers or the sophisticated urban teaching hospitals. A fact of American life is that medicine has been and still remains a middle-class institution.

Of course, physicians serve the poor and practice in underprivileged areas, but have they really been trained to concentrate on taking care of the middle class? In this chapter we will describe, but not defend, the medical care system (or the sickness system) that exists in this country today. There are four medical institutional elements that are related; and there is one additional element that impacts on the institutional components. I refer to this element as the "community." These different components or elements of the system will be examined.

THE SYSTEM'S GOALS

Before examining each of the components in detail, it is appropriate to keep in mind the general goals of our nation's health care system. These goals are presently being met in varying degrees, depending on the geographic locale and the economic status of the individual. Some of the gaps in the medical care system are seen when the goals are weighed against what is actually happening in the medical care world. In short, the traditional American medical system has aimed at the following goals:

- The system should be available to all the people.
- The system should be both psychologically and socially acceptable to all those using it.
- The system should have quality.
- The system should be comprehensive and stress maximum economy.

While these goals are noble, they still need to be weighed against some fundamental questions such as:

- What place and importance should be given to health care in managing our political and social systems?
- What kind of a life is it appropriate to expect medicine to help us achieve?
- How much and what kind of health does a society need in order to be a good society?
- Who is to provide this health care, pay for it, and take responsibility for it?

Given these goals and questions, let us examine the various components of the medical care system.

OUTREACH ELEMENT

The first component of the medical care system is the outreach element. In essence, the traditional system attempts to meet the patient's primary medical care needs through outreach programs. These programs are generally decentralized. They are scattered activities. Outreach activities include private physicians' offices in the community, health care centers, group practices, ambulatory care arrangements, and outpatient activities of health maintenance organizations (HMOs), among other activities.

Traditionally, most patients in America have received care through their primary care physician (or the solo practitioner). This is the most common example of the system's outreach component. Private or solo practitioners provide the bulk of the American outreach activity. At the same time, the urban poor may use city health clinics, public health nurses, or visiting nurses associations. The outreach element also includes groups like school nurses, sophisticated group practices that are free-standing from hospitals, the myriad of storefront clinic arrangements that are found in urban centers, and the multispecialty offices in the inner city called "Medicaid mills" that proliferate in some of our urban areas. Other social agencies have from time to time been involved in the outreach component. Churches often are involved in screening activities and in providing centers for referral through physicians or hospitals. This outreach phase is the beginning of the referral sequence for many patients in our present medical care system.

In the outreach component we are able to distinguish easily two classes of care. As we have noted, one type of care is offered to the middle-class consumers, the other is given to the poor. These two groups take different routes in the outreach element. The middle class historically has been served by the private practitioner and the primary care physician. Presently, there are 600,000 physicians or 240 physicians per 100,000 population.[2] However, there are slightly over 70,000 general practitioners, of which 46,000 specialize in family practice and 24,000 are in general practice.[3]

The record shows that there is a maldistribution of physicians; urban areas and large parts of the inner city as well as our depressed rural areas have a paucity of physicians. Rarely do you find members of the middle class using city health clinics, neighborhood health centers, or mental health program clinics. It is much more common for the medically indigent to use these sites. The real and significant difference between the two populations is how the middle class and the poor class are referred into the medical institutions in the system. Clearly, the two groups are not referred with the same social and psychological acceptance. Thus, the outreach component of our traditional system is in trouble. Indeed, an increasing problem is that the middle class is also having difficulty being referred into the other sectors of the medical care system. Witness the growth in physician referral programs used by numerous hospitals as a service and marketing technique. Even middle-class patients now have some difficulty finding primary care practitioners in their quiet suburban areas. Simply put, many middle-class consumers cannot guide themselves through the medical care system. The patients want physicians to take care of the whole person, not just the orthopedic, urologic, or psychiatric problem. This new problem for the middle class is the same one that our poor have experienced for years, conveniences and accessibility of quality care. Now that the entire system, and especially the outreach component, is coming under attack, perhaps there will be a change.

OUTPATIENT ELEMENT

The second component of our health system is the outpatient component. This is the part of the system that embodies the traditional hospital clinics and outpatient services. Historically, the clinics located in large urban areas were created for teaching purposes or to service the poor. The outpatient element also embraces the traditional hospital emergency departments and the two hybrid services, walk-in services and trauma services. It also includes the ambulance squads, emergency medical technicians (EMTs), the municipal policeman and fireman, and the suburban community ambulance services. In addition, hospital-based group practices are included in this element.

In analyzing the outpatient component we have to recognize that there are differences between hospital clinics. Those that are associated with large medical centers and teaching hospitals are used primarily for teaching purposes and are usually staffed with medical students and residents. Community hospital clinics, on the other hand, may be staffed with active attending physicians and are intended primarily for providing service. The continued need to train physicians and other medical practitioners will ensure the need for teaching clinics. Generally, the service clinics have been more acceptable for patients than the teaching clinics.

The most interesting aspect of the outpatient component is the emergency department. Studies have shown that more than 60 percent of all emergency cases that visit emergency departments are not true clinical emergencies. This is further evidence of the problem of access in our medical care system.

Why do so many patients use the emergency department? If we trace the evolution of the emergency department, we see that the volume began to increase sharply after World War II, and it has continued to grow steadily since that time. The emergency departments remain the one marketplace of medical care where there is an interface between the middle class and the poor. Both groups accept this service. There is no stigma in going to an emergency department. But there is definitely a stigma attached to waiting on a hard wooden bench in a teaching clinic in one of our large urban medical centers.These clinics are the embodiment of the two-class system but there is change and improvement taking place. Many large teaching hospitals in urban centers find themselves serving a disproportionate number of poor and older citizens. Serious questions are being raised about the future of university teaching clinics as many of these teaching clinics reorganize into private and group practice arrangements.

There are very few financial barriers in going to the emergency department. It is open for emergencies, urgent care, and other routine services and is not primarily interested in a patient's ability to pay. This is to the credit of the hospitals who sponsor them. It is not unusual to see an executive sitting next to a welfare recipient in a busy city emergency department. This is the one place in the outpatient component that has served to "bandage the gap" in the health care delivery system. But this is not enough.

Ambulance services are an outpatient activity that has taken on increased status with the advent of paramedics, cardiopulmonary resuscitation teams, and electronic monitoring. However, for millions who live in cities there are still two kinds of ambulance services. One is the municipal service, which is really an extension of the police ambulance or fire department. The other is the community ambulance staffed primarily for the people who can afford ambulances. This is another example of the two-class system.

INPATIENT ELEMENT

The third element is the inpatient (hospital) component. This is represented and characterized by the hospital bed. We have come to accept the hospital as synonymous with the bed. Over the last decade there has been a significant change in the types of beds. The number of general medical/surgical beds has decreased as the number of intensive care beds has increased. Hospitals continue to use the bed as the benchmark of occupancy, service, and financing, yet only 10 percent of the health needs of the patients in our system are cared for in the inpatient part of the hospital.

The general hospitals in this country can be classified into two clinical groups: teaching hospitals and community hospitals. Despite a major overlap between the two groups, the major teaching hospital is a different species from the community hospital. Each type has its own needs and offers something different. Their organizations are basically quite different. Time will tell which type of hospital has the most potential for change and improvement for the system.

The difficulties that are inherent in the hospital system stem from the dependency on the hospital bed. For example, one model of the economy of hospitals indicates that hospitals are controlled by their medical staff who seek to maximize their own income and in so doing use the hospital bed extensively, which begins the vicious circle of increased hospital cost. As it now stands, the economics of the hospital bed requires that the bed be filled for the hospital to stay solvent. The present inpatient system has a great deal of overlapping coverage or duplication of services. This is why mergers, shared services, and linkages are now in vogue and will undoubtedly increase and become more common. This trend may be one step toward improving care as well as toward holding a line on costs. Still, hospitals will need to strive for productivity, quality, and better bottom lines through efficiency.

An interesting phenomenon in the inpatient system is that physicians are regarded by hospitals as both consumers and providers. Under this model, hospitals provide facilities not for the patient, but for the physicians who admit the patients. In turn, the physicians provide care to their patients and are therefore themselves providers. Understanding this arrangement is critical in identifying the control valve in the cost of medical care.

EXTENDED ELEMENT

The fourth element in the system is the extended component. Included in this area are such things as long-term care hospitals, home care programs, skilled nursing facilities (SNFs), intermediate care facilities (ICFs), custodial care situations, boarding homes or personal care residences, durable medical equipment companies, visiting nurses, hospice care, wellness programs, freestanding oncology centers, birthing centers, independent laboratories, rehabilitation centers, and certain other specialty hospitals.

The scientific, professional component that has done such a magnificent job in our inpatient facilities seems to be lagging in the treatment provided in our skilled nursing facilities and in many of the other extended care programs. The extended component seems to receive relatively little support and therefore might deteriorate and become the weakest link in the system. As an illustration, one has only to look at the deplorable conditions of many of our nation's boarding homes.

COMMUNITY ELEMENT

The fifth and final element is noninstitutional. This is the community component. The community can be viewed from multiple perspectives. The first is a view of the community as a consumer group, those who use health care facilities. Today, consumers are better educated than ever about health care and are an active group. They are concerned over such issues as the right to die and living wills. This is illustrated by the well-known Karen Ann Quinlan and Nancy Cruzan cases, which raised ethical and moral questions regarding medical care and the patients' and families' rights.

The community element also includes health manpower resources, that is, the medical training programs in our medical schools and in our teaching hospitals. Aligned to this manpower element are the labor unions. Unions in this sense are seen not as third-party payers but as representatives of manpower resources. They are a major force in the supply and demand function for labor. The second perspective embraces the community and its demographic shifts. The aging of America as well as new diseases like AIDS will also affect our hospitals' long-range plans.

Finally, there is the role of the federal and state governments as part of the community component. In this context, we must consider the dollars that are spent on health care through the federal government. Americans spend billions on health care yearly, with much of this expenditure through Medicare and Medicaid programs.

Apart from these aspects, the community element also includes private insurance plans and health maintenance organizations, as well as other types of managed health care programs. Also included in this community element are life style changes and the rapid rise in technology. Beyond this, there are also within the community component educational and health environmental programs such as pollution control. Finally, in the community component we must include the politics of health care.

In summary, the American medical care system can be viewed as having the best and worst in a medical care system. From this examination, one thing is clear, improvements are needed. There is the need for some reform. That is a challenge for all of us. But there is one thing we can count on, that the medical institutional elements of our system will continue to change in response to the ever-changing community needs.

NOTES

1. *Webster's New World Dictionary of the American Language,* College Edition (Cleveland and New York: The World Publishing Co., 1958), p. 1480.
2. I. Donald Snook, Jr., *Opportunities on Health and Medical Careers* (Lincolnwood, Ill.: VGM Career Horizons, 1991), p. 22.
3. *Physician Characteristics and Distribution in the U.S.,* 1990 Ed.

Appendix A

GLOSSARY

Accreditation. A process used by the Joint Commission on Accreditation of Healthcare Organizations (JCAHO) to evaluate the quality of patient care at hospitals and health facilities. [22]

Accredited Hospital. A hospital which meets specific operating standards set by the Joint Commission on Accreditation of Healthcare Organizations (JCAHO) or by the American Osteopathic Association. Typically, the Seal of Accreditation is displayed in the lobby of a hospital. [22]

Admission. The formal acceptance of inpatients into a hospital or other inpatient health facility. Such inpatients are typically provided with room, board, and continuous nursing service and stay at least over night. [2, 8]

Admitting Department. The hospital department which secures patient demographic and financial information on inpatients for registration purposes; schedules pre-admission testing; coordinates patient room assignments; records all patient movement including transfers and discharges for the purpose of maintaining accurate census data; and disseminates patient information to other hospital departments. (Synonym: Admissions Office) [8]

Advertising. The act or practice of attracting public attention with the specific intent of generating interest or inducing purchase. Advertising paid for and generally placed in the mass media. [23]

Agency Contract Nurse. A service referred to as an outside agency which contracts with hospitals to provide registered nurses, licensed practical nurses, and nursing assistants. (Synonym: Rent-A-Nurse Company) [10]

NOTE: The numbers [in brackets] at the end of each definition denote the chapter(s) in which the term, word, or phrase is first introduced or primarily used.

Alliance. A formal agreement between several hospitals and/or hospital systems for specific purposes. These arrangements usually operate under a set of bylaws or other written regulations. [3]

Allied Health Professional. A health worker other than a physician, dentist, podiatrist, or nurse who is specially trained, and in some cases, licensed, e.g., a physician's assistant. Depending upon the hospital or health facility, this individual may perform tasks that could be performed by a physician. An allied health professional always works under the supervision of a health professional. [9]

Ambulatory Care. Medical or health services provided on an outpatient basis. It usually implies the patients are ambulatory and came to the facility for a specific outpatient treatment or service. (Synonym: Outpatient Care) [1]

Ambulatory Care Center, Free standing. A facility, not on a hospital campus, offering medical, surgical, diagnostic, and rehabilitative care on an outpatient basis. [6]

Ambulatory Hospital. A program based in the hospital or other institution offering intensive medical, psychiatric, nursing, or rehabilitative services to patients during the day hours. [6]

Ambulatory Surgery, Hospital. Minor elective surgical procedures provided by a hospital on an outpatient basis. By admitting and discharging patients on the day of surgery, such programs reduce hospital costs. (Synonyms: Short Procedures Unit (SPU), Same Day Surgery, Come and Go Surgery, and Outpatient Surgery) [2, 6]

Ambulatory Surgical Facility, Freestanding. A facility, physically and/or geographically separate and apart from the hospital, which provides surgical treatment to outpatients who do not require overnight hospitalization. Note: Surgical procedures done in offices of private physicians or dentists are not included in this category unless such offices have a distinct area that is used solely for outpatient surgical treatment on a routine, organized basis. (Synonyms: Freestanding Surgi-Center, Surgi-Center) [6]

American College of Healthcare Executives (ACHE). 840 North Lakeshore Drive, Chicago, Illinois 60611. Formed in 1933. Professional society for hospital and healthcare managers and executives. It was formerly called the American College of Hospital Administrators (ACHA). The name was changed in 1985.

American Hospital Association (AHA). 840 N. Lake Shore Drive, Chicago, Illinois 60611. Formed in 1898. A nationwide association which promotes the public's welfare through the development of better hospital care for all people. The AHA conducts research and educational programs in areas of health care administration, hospital economics, hospital facilities and design, and community relations. In addition, the AHA represents hospitals as a national spokesman for legislation. The AHA has several separate professional divisions; for example, American Academy of Hospital Attorneys, American Society for Hospital Central Service Personnel. The AMA also offers policy guidance to governmental agencies. [9]

American Medical Association (AMA). 535 Dearborn Street, Chicago, Illinois 60610. Formed in 1847. A nationwide professional association of licensed physicians. Action: Monitors the quality of medical practice. The AMA provides information on drugs, medical therapy, research, food and nutrition, cosmetics and medical quackery; determines the conditions of medical practice and payment; and acts as a watchdog over the growing governmental interest in the nations health. The AMA also offers policy guidance to governmental agencies. [9]

Ancillary Services. Therapeutic or diagnostic services provided by specific hospital departments (other than nursing service) including but not limited to x-ray, laboratories, and anesthesiology. Other (electrocardiograms) ancillary services include but are not limited to respiratory therapy, electroencephalography, heart station, rehabilitative medicine, and pharmacy. [11]

Anesthesiology. The branch of medicine that deals with the administration and study of anesthetics. It involves the administration of local, general, or regional anesthesia before and during surgery. [11]

Anesthesiology Department. That hospital department staffed by anesthesiologists and nurse anesthetists who administer anesthesia and anesthetics to patients so that surgical or other authorized procedures may be performed. [11]

Annual Report. A yearly publication prepared and issued by a hospital which details the state of the institution's operations and financial position. Typically, the year's accomplishments are highlighted, as well as its future plans and programs. [23]

Audit Medical and Patient Care. A periodic and systematic review of quality care within a hospital usually done by a committee or a designated person following a set process. [20]

Average Census. The average number of patients—both inpatients and an equivalent number of inpatients—who receive medical or nursing care during a specific reporting period (typically one year or month). [17]

Average Daily Census. The average number of inpatients receiving care each day during a reporting period, excluding newborns. [12]

Baccalaureate Degree Program, Nursing. A formal program of study in a four-year college or university which educates students in the nursing field. Typically, the college's nursing school provides both classroom and laboratory teaching. The college's own or its affiliated hospital provides the clinical teaching. Upon graduation from the program, individuals are awarded a bachelor of arts or bachelor or science degree in nursing. Graduates are then eligible to take the state nursing examinations for licensure as registered nurses. (Synonym: Bachelor of Science in Nursing, BSN) [10]

Bad Debt. An account which is uncollectible from a patient, although the patient has or may have the ability to pay. This results in a credit loss for the hospital, clinic, or other health care facility. These losses may be reflected as an allowance from revenue or as an expense of doing business of the entity. [2, 17]

Balance Sheet. A summary listing of an institution's assets, liabilities, and net worth showing the financial condition of the hospital or business at a specific point in time. For hospitals, net worth is commonly referred to as the fund balance. [17]

Bed. A bed located in a hospital or nursing home used for inpatients. Beds are used as one important measure of an institution's capacity and size. [2]

Bed Allocation Policy. A hospital's method of assigning inpatient beds. A hospital may establish its own policy. Policies may be established to maximize occupancy or hospital resources; segregate clinical areas—medicine, surgery, obstetrics, and gynecology; minimize bad debts or maximize revenue; and/or to support the hospital's teaching programs (interns and residents) by assigning beds according to teaching needs. [8]

Bed Size. The number of hospital beds, vacant or occupied, maintained regularly for use by inpatients during a reporting period. (The typical reporting period is 12 months.) To determine this amount, first add the total number of beds which are available every day during the hospital's reporting period. Then, divide this amount by the total number of days in the reporting period. (Synonym: Statistical Beds) [2]

Bedside Telemonitoring Equipment. A sophisticated piece of medical equipment used at a patient's bedside for a variety of functions, including recording electrocardiograms, measuring heart and respiratory rates, and recording blood pressure. Although such monitors are equipped with easy-to-use indicators and controls, only medical/nursing personnel who are trained to use the monitor should be responsible for its proper use. [10]

Beeper System. That communications system that medical and health care professionals often use to enable them to stay in touch with the hospital or their office staff. Beeper systems are the name given to the radio wave pagers. They can be digital, voice or a combination of both. Within the hospital, the paging system or beeper system is usually coordinated through the telephone office. [15]

Blood Bank. A medical laboratory which collects and types blood from donors, then refrigerates the blood until it is needed for transfusions. The unit also analyzes blood from donors to determine compatibility. This process is referred to as "typing" and "crossmatching." [11]

Blood Bank Technologist. A trained individual, working under the direction of a laboratory director, physician, or pathologist, whose responsibilities include collecting, classifying, storing, and processing of blood, as well as preparing components from whole blood, detecting and identifying antibodies in blood from patients and donors, and selecting and delivering blood suitable for transfusion. [11]

Blue Cross (BC). A private insurance plan which provides coverage for the insured for hospital costs. Most Blue Cross subscribers sign up for coverage at their workplace under a group plan. [8, 16]

Board Certified. A professional title of considerable merit awarded to a physician who passes examinations administered by the professional organization which regulates his/her specialty. The examination cannot be taken until the physician meets requirements established by the specialty board, making him/her board eligible. [9]

Board of Trustees. *See* Governing Body.

Bond Ratings. General measurements of a bond's quality provided to guide investors in making investments. Bonds which are rated Aaa/AAA are judged to be of the best quality because they carry the smallest degree of investment risk. Bonds are generally rated by one of two companies: Standard and Poors, or Moodys. [17]

Brand Name Drug. The registered trademark which a manufacturer assigns to one of its drug products. Note: A drug's brand name differs from a drug's generic name, which is the official name by which the drug is known scientifically. Drugs are advertised to physicians chiefly by brand name. (Many states have an antisubstitution law which forbids a pharmacist from substituting a physician's prescription for a brand name drug with either an equivalent brand name drug or a generic drug made by a different manufacturer even though either of the substitutions may be less expensive than the prescribed drugs.) (Synonyms: Trade Name, Patent Name) [12]

Budget. The dollar amounts required to meet a hospital's immediate administrative objectives, as well as its operation and financing plans for a given time period, usually a year. It is the hospital's plan for that time period expressed in dollars and cents. [17]

Budget, Cash. The details of a business or hospital's anticipated receipts and cash disbursements for a forthcoming budget period. It is usually used to forecast the need for cash to meet operating expenses and to determine the amount of cash that will be available for capital purchases, acquisitions, and investing. [17]

Business Office Manager. That individual who supervises and coordinates the operations of a hospital's business office, including the supervision of office functions, such as bookkeeping, typing, clerical services, word processing, record keeping, files, and reports in accordance with hospital standards. [17]

Bylaws. The rules, regulations, and ordinances enacted by a given organization to provide the basis for its own self-government. In a hospital, two major sets of bylaws are the governing body bylaws, or hospital bylaws, and the medical staff bylaws. [4, 9]

Capital Budget. A financial plan detailing anticipating capital expenditures principally for equipment (medical and non-medical) and building renovation and construction. The sources of these funds are identified as part of the capital budget. Potential sources are operating funds, restricted funds, and outside financing such as leases or debt finances and fund raising. [17]

Cardiac Coronary Care Unit (CCU). A specialized cardiac unit reserved for observation and recovery of patients who have undergone an intensive cardiac procedure or who have critical cardiac problems (e.g., heart attacks). Units are equipped with electrocardiographic and hemodynamic monitoring equipment. [10]

Certification. The process by which a government or private agency or a health related association evaluates and recognizes individual, institutional, or educational programs in meeting predetermined standards. [22]

Certified Laboratory Assistant (CLA). Individuals who perform routine clinical laboratory procedures and work under the supervision of a medical technologist or pathologist. [11]

Chief Executive Officer (CEO). The individual responsible for the overall management of the hospital. An individual appointed by the governing body to assure that the mission and goals of the institution are carried out as determined by the bylaws of the hospital. The job includes planning, organizing and directing all hospital activities in accordance with objectives and policies established by the board, developing ongoing and future hospital programs, presenting annual budgets, planning and implementing sound organizational plans. (Synonyms: Administrator, President, Hospital Administrator, Hospital Director, Superintendent) [2, 3, 5]

Chief Financial Officer (CFO). The individual responsible for an organization's overall financial plans and policies along with the administration of accounting practices. The job includes directing the hospital's treasury, budgeting, audit, tax, and accounting functions and may include the purchase of real estate. Specific responsibilities include developing and coordinating all necessary and appropriate accounting and statistical data with and for all the departments. [18]

Chief Operating Officer (COO). The second highest management position in the hospital. He/she is responsible for the management of day-to-day internal hospital operations. In the absence of the chief executive officer, the chief operating officer is responsible for managing the hospital. (Synonyms: Assistant Administrator, Executive Vice-President, Senior Vice-President) [2, 5]

Children's Hospital. This is a specialty hospital, specializing in inpatient and outpatient care limited to the treatment of diseases and injuries of children. [2]

Chronic Illness. Any illness that has continued for a long period of time and may recur in the future. Alterations in such illnesses are slow. [1]

Clinic. An independent organization of physicians and allied health personnel or a hospital operated facility designed to provide preventive, diagnostic, therapeutic, rehabilitative, or palliative services on an outpatient basis. [6]

Clinical Engineer. A professional with an associate or bachelor of science degree in biomedical engineering. This individual utilizes engineering techniques to repair or develop equipment, instruments, processes, and systems for the medical care of patients and the overall maintenance and improvement of health care systems. Some biomedical engineers develop lasers, pacemakers, and artificial organs such as hearts and kidneys. Others adapt computer systems to hospital systems to increase operating efficiency. Typically, they work in hospitals or private medically related industries or medical settings. (Synonym: Biomedical Engineer) [14]

Clinical Nurse Specialist. A registered nurse with both a master's degree and clinical expertise in a clinical area (e.g., surgical, critical care, medicine, or cardiology). [10]

Clinical Outcomes. A form of medical and/or nursing evaluation involving the measurement of the patient care process against criteria such as the status of the patient at discharge. [20]

Community Hospital. A hospital that is established to meet the medical and health needs of a specific geographic area. Usually these hospitals are nonprofit but may be proprietary for profit. Community hospitals are generally nonfederal, short-term, and general care hospitals. [2,12]

Comprehensive Outpatient Rehabilitation Facility (CORF). A facility providing comprehensive outpatient rehabilitation services, including physician's services, physical therapy, occupational therapy, speech-language pathology, respiratory therapy, prosthetic supplies, and home environment evaluation. These services are reimbursable under Medicare Part B. [12]

Computerized Axial Tomography (CAT). A radiographic technique more sensitive than conventional x-ray systems in detecting variations among soft tissues with similar densities. It provides highly detailed, cross-sectional, three-dimensional pictures which, because they are thin slices or cross sections of the body, establish more precisely than conventional x-rays the area and depth of the abnormality. (Synonym: CAT Scan) [11]

Consent Forms. The documents that patients are asked to sign giving permission to the hospital or its physicians to perform procedures during the patient's hospital stay whether as an out-patient or in-patient. There are two general types of consent forms, one that details their general treatment and diagnosis and the other one for special medical or surgical procedures. The most important element in the issue of consent is that the physician in the hospital clearly explain the procedures to be performed to the patient and obtain the patient's consent to the procedures. This is known as an informal consent form. [8]

Continuing Medical Education (CME). Postgraduate education aimed at maintaining, updating, and extending a physician's knowledge and skills. Many professional organizations and state licensing boards require a physician to participate in CME activities. [9]

Contract Management. A system whereby hospital management contracts with an outside management company to provide certain management services, e.g., dietary, housekeeping, and data processing services. It is also possible to employ contract management for the total management of a hospital. (Synonym: Contract Service) [13,14]

Controller. The hospital position responsible for the traditional financial activities of the hospital, including general accounting, reimbursement, and budgeting. In smaller institutions, this position may also be the Chief Financial Officer (CFO). In larger institutions, the controller reports to a CFO. [18]

Corporate Restructuring. The regrouping of a hospital's corporate hierarchy by creating holding companies or foundations in order to guard assets, provide flexibility for diversification, accomplish a broader mission, increase effectiveness, and permit capital accumulation. (Synonym: Corporate Reorganization) [3]

Cost Reimbursement. Payment to hospitals and other providers by a third-party carrier for costs actually incurred by the providers; cost rates are calculated after the service is rendered. [16]

Cost Reports. The cost analysis documents prepared by a health care facility to be submitted to third-party payers as part of contract agreements. These reports are used as the basis for cost reimbursement. [16]

Credentials Committee. A committee of the medical staff that interviews and reviews credentials and delineation of privileges for each new medical staff applicant. [9, 20]

Darling Case. A landmark legal case, Darling v. Charleston Community Hospital, found that the hospital was responsible to oversee and monitor the quality and process of medical care in the institution and that these functions were not exclusively the responsibility of the medical staff. [4, 21]

Delinquent Medical Records. Those inpatient medical records not completed within a given time period, usually 15 to 30 days following the patient's discharge. [19]

Development Office. That section of the hospital responsible to direct, plan, and coordinate direct fundraising activities and programs for the hospital. This section may also be responsible for the hospital's public relations activities. (Synonym: Fundraising Office) [23]

Diagnostic Related Group (DRG) Rate. A dollar amount used by Medicare to pay hospitals for services rendered. It is based on the average of all patients belonging to a specific DRG adjusted for economic factors, inflation and bad debts. [1, 16]

Dietary Department. That hospital department equipped, designed and staffed to prepare food to meet the normal and therapeutic nutritional needs of the patients and hospital staff. (Synonym: Food Service Department) [13]

Dietician. A professional, educated and trained to deal with the scientific aspects of human nutrition and diets. The dietician develops specific food and nutritional plans for patients. [13]

Diploma School of Nursing. A three-year professional nursing program, generally affiliated with a hospital, which leads to a diploma. [10]

Discharge Planning. The planning and organization process undertaken by a committee of a hospital medical staff that addresses patient discharges into the community, home, or appropriate health care facilities. This process begins at the time of admission or, in elective cases, prior to admission. [13, 20]

Elective Admission. The admission of a patient to a hospital prior to the actual scheduled date of admission. This admission can be delayed without potential risk to the health of the individual. [8]

Electrocardiography (EKG). A cardiac procedure used at the heart station to diagnose irregularities in heart action. It records changes in electrical current during a heartbeat, providing an important source of medical diagnostic information.

Electroencephalography (EEG). A procedure used to measure the brain's electrical signals. This is useful in diagnosing epilepsy, brain tumors, strokes, and other metabolic abnormalities. [12]

Emergency Admission. The admission of a patient to a hospital immediately or within a very short period of time in order to save the patient's life or to protect the patient's health and well being. Other general categories of admission are urgent, usually requiring admission within 12–24 hours, or elective, when a patient can wait for admission without any adverse effects. [7, 8]

Emergency Center, Freestanding (FEC). A facility structured, equipped, and staffed to offer primary, urgent, and emergency services. These facilities often offer laboratory and radiographic services as well, and often have transfer agreements with area hospitals for sending severely ill patients needing hospitalization to the hospital once the patients are stable. [6]

Emergency Room (ER). That department or unit of a hospital organized to provide medical services necessary to sustain life or to prevent critical consequences. This area sometimes provides non-urgent, walk-in care. The department is usually staffed 24 hours per day by physicians and nurses. (Synonym: Emergency Department, Emergency Service) [7, 25]

Emergency Patient. An outpatient, usually acutely ill, who uses a hospital or free-standing emergency department for treatment. [7]

Executive Committee. The senior committee of a governing body (hospital board or medical staff). It may also be the ruling body. [9]

Expenses. The sum of all incurred costs for services used or consumed in performing some activity during a given time period and from which no benefit will exist beyond the stated period. [17]

Fiduciary. A person who undertakes a solemn duty to act for the benefit of another, under a given set of circumstances (e.g., the members of the governing body of a hospital have a fiduciary responsibility to the community). [4]

Financial Statements. Summaries of the financial activities of a hospital or other business. The balance sheet includes itemized listings of the hospital's assets and liabilities and the net worth of the hospital. The income statement, or profit and loss statement, lists the hospital's income or revenue and its expenses or costs. [17]

Fluoroscopy. Technique used to view the body structure by sending x-rays through the body part to be examined and then observing the shadows cast on a glaring screen. [11]

Formulary. A listing of drugs, usually by their generic names, intended to include sufficient range of medicines to enable a physician or dentist to prescribe medically appropriate treatment for all reasonable common illnesses. A formulatory may also be a listing of drugs for which a third party will or will not pay. [12]

Full Time Equivalent (FTE). The term used in hospital budgeting and human resources that represents the number of worked hours that a full-time employee would be expected to work in a given year. In other words, 40 hours a week or 2,080 annual hours. This term is used in hospital budgeting, position control and productivity.

General Fund/Fund Accounting. Technique that accounts for separate entities in a hospital fund. The account group used to record transactions arising out of general operations in the day-to-day financial and operational activities of the hospital. (Synonym: Hospital Accounting) [18]

Generic Drug. The official scientific name for a drug. [12]

Governing Body. A hospital's ruling body, responsible for the institution's overall operation. Its essential functions include defining objectives, mandating policies, maintaining the programs and resources necessary to implement policies, and monitoring progress to guarantee the policy objectives are met. In addition, it hires the hospital's CEO. Note: The Board of Trustees should not be mistaken for the Lay Advisory Board. (Synonyms: The Board, Board of Directors, Board of Trustees, Board of Governors) [4]

Graduate Nurse (GN). A nurse who has graduated from an approved program of professional nursing but who has not yet received the registered nurse (RN) licensure. [10]

Group Practice. A formal association of physicians providing either specialty or comprehensive medical care on an outpatient basis. (Synonyms: Single Specialty Group, General Practice Group, Multispecialty Group) [6]

Group Purchasing. An arrangement where more than one hospital, a group of hospitals, band together often through a third party, e.g., the group purchaser, in order to purchase goods and services at the lowest price because of quantity purchasing. (Synonym: Shared Purchasing) [15]

Head Nurse. The registered nurse responsible and accountable for the total operation of one single nursing unit 24 hours a day, seven days a week. The head nurse supervises the personnel in this patient care unit, is accountable for the quality of the nursing care on the unit, controls the supplies and material for the unit, and usually schedules the nursing staff in the unit. Generally, head nurses have a staff of nurses working for them. (Synonym: Nurse Manager, Patient Care Manager) [3, 10]

Health Administration. The management of resources, procedures, and systems operating to meet the needs and wants of a health care system. (Synonyms: Health Care Administration, Hospital Administration) [5]

Health System. The organization of human resources, facilities, and medical technology. (Synonym: Medical System) [20]

Health Maintenance Organization (HMO). There are two fundamental types of HMO plans: (1) the group model, where HMOs contract with several group practices and share the risk of the venture with the physicians; and (2) Independent Practice Associations (IPAs), lose-knit, prepaid plans that contract with individual physicians to treat patients in their offices, often on a fee-for-service basis. [16]

Heart Station. That unit or section of a hospital that coordinates cardiac tests and procedures. Some may be done on an outpatient basis (e.g., EKGs). [11, 12]

Hill-Burton Act. The legislative act which led to federal legislation and programs offering federal support for construction and modernization of hospitals and other health facilities. This program began with Public Law 79-725, The Hospital Survey and Construction Act of 1946, and has been amended frequently. [1]

Home Care Nurse. A registered nurse (preferably with a BSN and two years of hospital experience) who intermittently visits patients at their home to carry out a nursing care plan approved by a physician. Typical duties include injections, incision care, rehabilitation activities, patient education, and other skilled care. (Synonym: Visiting Nurse) [10]

Home Health Care. A formal program offering medical and nursing care, therapeutic services, and social services to patients in their homes. (Synonym: Home Care Services) [10, 13]

Hospice Care. A program providing palliative and supportive care for terminally ill patients and their families either directly or on a consulting basis with the patient's physician or another community agency. Emphasis is placed on system control, preparation for death, and support of the survivors. A hospice program may be housed and based in a facility such as a hospital or a freestanding hospice. [25]

Hospital. An institution producing medical and health care every day around the clock. Its primary function is to provide inpatient and outpatient services, including diagnostic and therapeutic services, for a variety of medical and surgical conditions. Some also provide emergency care. Hospitals can be teaching or nonteaching, specialty or nonspecialty (psychiatric, general, etc.), owned or not-for-profit (government, local, private) entities. The majority of hospitals in the United States are short-term, general, and nonprofit. [1]

Hospital Bylaws. The guidelines, rules, and regulations governing the actions and regulating the affairs of a hospital governing board. [4]

Hospital Chaplains. Members of the clergy who provide religious minister and pastoral care and services to patients, their families, and members of the hospital staff. [13]

Hospital Information System (HIS). A system which collects data from many areas of a hospital to provide all levels of hospital management with timely, meaningful information on hospital operation. [18]

Hospital Ledger. An accounting record detailing the various accounts in a hospital categorized into assets, liabilities, revenues, and expenses. Entries are made into this document periodically (generally monthly) from various journals. The general ledger allows for financial analysis over a long period of time. [18]

Human Resources. The hospital department responsible for, in conjunction with other hospital departments, recruitment, selection, orientation, and employee training programs. The department is also responsible for maintaining personnel records and statistics, initiating and maintaining salary and wage administration, and recommending personnel policy and procedure to the hospital administrator. (Synonym: Personnel Department) [15]

Incident Report. A written report detailing an accident or error in the care of a patient. Hospitals require the nurse and/or the physician in charge to complete the form as soon as possible following the accident to ensure accuracy. (Synonym: Accident Report) [21]

Income Statement of Revenue and Expenses. A summary of the operations of a hospital in terms of revenue generated from patient services and other sources and the expenses incurred to render those services. (Synonym: Profit and Loss Statement, Income Statement) [17]

Independent Laboratory. A freestanding laboratory not affiliated with any physician's office or hospital. [25]

Infection Control. The process of identification, control, and prevention of hospital-acquired (nosocomial) infections. This is usually a responsibility of a hospital medical staff committee in conjunction with and with the support of an infection control practitioner. [14]

Infection Control Committee. That hospital or medical staff committee responsible for overseeing the infection control activities in the institution. The committee usually consists of representatives from the medical staff, the clinical laboratory, administration, nursing staff, and, at times, the housekeeping department. [14, 20]

Informed Consent. Consent given by a patient for a proposed medical treatment or procedure after a physician has explained the treatment or procedure, the risks involved, as well as alternatives available which a reasonable person would consider material to decision making. [19]

Inpatient. A patient who has been admitted for at least one night to a hospital or other health facility for the purpose of receiving diagnostic treatment or other medical service. [6]

Inpatient Component. An element of the hospital-medical care system characterized by the hospital bed. (Synonym: Hospital Component) [25]

Intensive Care Unit (ICU). A special medical and nursing section of a hospital with extensive monitoring and treatment equipment allowing minute-to-minute observation and treatment of critically ill or injured patients. [10]

Intermediate Care Facility (ICF). An institution or distinct part of an institution providing nursing care or rehabilitative services to patients who do not require inpatient hospital care. [10]

Intern. A graduate of a medical or dental school enrolled in the first year of postgraduate education in an accredited training program, usually in a hospital. (Synonym: Post-Graduate Year, First-Year Resident) [9]

Internship (Medical). A period of "on-the-job" training for physicians and other health professionals usually lasting one year after graduation from medical school. [9]

Investor-Owned Hospital. A privately owned medical facility operating for profit. (Synonym: Proprietary Hospital) [2]

Job Description. A summary of the key features, elements, or requirements of a specific job category. This summary is generally written after a review of the job, called a job analysis. [15]

Joint Commission of the Accreditation of Health Care Organizations (JCAHO). 875 N. Michigan Avenue, Chicago, Illinois 60611. Formed in 1951. A private, nonprofit organization that traces its beginnings to the American College of Surgeons but now involves other professional associations including the American Hospital Association, the American Medical Association and the American College of Physicians. Its purpose is to establish minimum standards of quality care and operations for hospitals. Hospitals voluntarily request a survey for accreditation. Most hospitals seek it since many other issues such as state licensure, third-party reimbursement, internships and residencies as well as expansion of facilities are contingent upon receiving accreditation. [22]

Joint Venture. An organization or association formed by two or more parties for a single purpose or undertaking. Such an organization may make its membership liable for the organization's debts. [3]

Laboratory Department. That unit or department in a hospital or health care facility staffed, equipped, and designed to perform clinical tests and procedures through detailed analysis and examination of specimens. The laboratory is usually divided into sections, including Anatomical Pathology, Clinical Chemistry, Cytopathology, Hematology and Microbiology. (Synonyms: Clinical Laboratory, Laboratory Service, Medical Laboratory, Laboratory, or Lab [11]

Laboratory Report. A document identifying the results of diagnostic tests in a clinical laboratory. Such reports, requested by a physician, are generally used to determine baseline clinical data on a patient or to determine a patient's diagnosis. [11]

Length of Stay (LOS). The length an inpatient stays in a hospital or other health facility from date of admission to date of discharge. [2]

Length of Stay, Average. The average number of days of service rendered to each patient who is discharged during a given time period. To compute this figure, divide the total number of days spent in the hospital by patients discharged in a given time period by the total number of inpatients discharged during the time period. Example: 120 total patients days for 20 patients discharged. The average length of stay is 120/20 = 6 days. [2]

Licensure. Permission granted to an individual or organization by competent authority, usually public, enabling the individual or organization to engage in a practice, occupation, or activity that, without permission, is unlawful. [10, 22]

Long-Range Plan. A corporate or managerial plan for the operation and functioning of a hospital or institution for the long term, usually three to ten years, including any planned changes in services to be provided, service areas, and proposed buildings or remodeling plans. (Synonym: Corporate Strategy) [24]

Long-Term Care. Health and medical care and social services provided on a continual basis to patients suffering from chronic medical and mental conditions. [2]

Long-Term Care Facilities. A range of institutions that provide various levels of long-term care including maintenance and/or nursing care to people who are unable to care for themselves, many of whom have health problems ranging from minimal to severe. Such facilities primarily provide care for patients with long-term illnesses or low prospects for recovery, who require regular medical assessment and continuous nursing care. This term includes freestanding institutions or other identifiable components of health care facilities providing nursing care and related services, as well as personal care and residential care. (Synonyms: Nursing Home, Intermediate Care Facilities, Skilled Nursing Facilities) [10]

Magnetic Resonance Imaging (MRI). A diagnostic procedure using large magnets and radio signals to produce tomographic images of a patient's anatomical structures. This diagnostic tool also has the capability of evaluating a patient's chemical disturbances at the cellular level. The older (original) term for this was Nuclear Magnetic Resonance (NMR). [11]

Mainframe. The central processing unit (CPU) of the computer system. (Synonym: Macro System) [18]

Maintenance Department. That unit, division or department in a hospital responsible for repair and servicing of a hospital's physical plant including the hospital grounds, buildings, and equipment. It may also include the provision, distribution, and monitoring of water, light, heat, power, and other building service systems throughout the physical plant. [14]

Malpractice. The professional misconduct or lack of ordinary skill in the performance of a professional act. A professional is liable for the damages or injuries caused by his/her malpractice. When applied to a health practitioner, it is called medical malpractice. [21]

Malpractice Suit. Legal proceeding by a plaintiff seeking enforcement of his rights for malpractice. [21]

Market Research. The planning, obtaining, display, and analysis of data related to the marketing of a product/service to fulfill a company's mission and objectives. [23]

Marketing. A system of planning, promoting, and distributing needed and wanted services to both present and potential customers. A hospital's customers can include physicians, patients, insurance companies, or employers. [23]

Marketing Audit. A marketing tool providing an extensive view of a hospital's or a business' services, its image, and its market segments. [23]

Marketing Plan/Program. The process of presenting products/services to the marketplace including product definition, product location or place, product price, and product promotion, including public relations and advertising. [23]

Medicaid "Mill." A place where physicians and other health practitioners continually diagnose and treat a large number of medically indigent patients, usually in an urban poverty area. These "mills" are characterized by a high number of patient visits and generally rapid care. They are not required to meet all the licensing and regulating requirements of a hospital, and thus may be a source of competition to a hospital's outpatient activities. [25]

Medicaid (MA). A federal health insurance plan, authorized by Title XIX of the Social Security Act, Public Law 89-97, administered by individual states to provide health care for the poor. (Synonym: Medical Assistance Program) [1, 2]

Medical College Admission Test (MCAT). A standardized test required or strongly recommended by nearly all American medical schools as part of the admission process. Results of this test are evaluated by the medical schools' admissions committees to determine a student's ability to handle medical school course work. [9]

Medical Director. The physician on the hospital medical staff who is either appointed by the board, elected by the medical staff, or employed by the institution to serve as the medical administrative head of medical staff affairs. If a physician is elected by the medical staff, he/she may be called the President of the Medical Staff. (Synonym: Chief of Staff) [9]

Medical Office Building (MOB). A building either freestanding or attached to a hospital where a physician or other health practitioner can establish an office. An MOB is sometimes used as a marketing tool for hospitals to attract and retain physicians. [6]

Medical Record. A patient file containing sufficient information to clearly identify the patient, to justify the patient's diagnosis and treatment, and to accurately document the results. The record serves as a basis for planning and continuity of patient care and provides a means of communication among physicians and any other professionals involved in the patient's care. The record also serves as a basis for review, study, and evaluation on serving and protecting the legal interests of the patient, hospital, and responsible practitioner. The content of each record is usually confidential. The record is the property of the hospital; however, others may have access to the record with signed release from the patient. (Synonym: Chart, Medical Chart) [19]

Medical Records, Department of. That hospital department responsible for the cataloging, maintenance, processing, and control of patient hospital medical records. This unit may be responsible for the statistical and qualitative preparation and analysis of the information in the medical record to aid in the evaluation of patient care. The department prepares records subpoenaed by the courts and interprets medical-legal aspects of records to protect the interests of the hospital. [19]

Medical School. An institution for higher learning accredited by the Association of American Medical Colleges. Medical colleges are accredited to provide courses in arts and science of medicine and related subjects and are empowered to grant an academic degree in medicine. [9]

Medical Staff, Attending. A category of a hospital's medical staff including physicians and dentists, who contribute actively to the hospital by admitting and caring for patients on a regular basis. The medical staff might also include other practitioners including podiatrists. These individuals are eligible to vote and hold office in the medical staff organization. [9]

Medical Staff Appointment. The appointment by the Hospital Board of Trustees of a physician or dentist to a hospital's medical staff based on the approval of the credentials committee of the medical staff. Appointment includes delineation of clinical privileges. There are different categories of medical staff membership: active, courtesy, consulting, and honorary. [4, 9]

Medical Staff Bylaws. A document required by the Joint Commission on the Accreditation of Hospitals Healthcare Organizations (JCAHO) outlining the activities, functions, roles, purpose, rules, and regulations of a hospital's medical staff. The bylaws identify and define the key operating committees of the medical staff and their functions. [9]

Medical Students. Individuals enrolled in an accredited medical school studying to become physicians. [9]

Medical Technologist. An individual trained in the use of clinical laboratory equipment to test human body tissues and fluids, culture bacteria to identify organisms causing disease, analyze blood factors, and trace cancer with radionuclides. Medical technologists specialize in blood banking microbiology, chemistry, and nuclear medical technology.

Medicare. Title XVIII of the Social Security Act, Public Law 89-97. A federal program that pays providers for certain medical and other health services for individuals 65 years of age or older or the disabled, regardless of their income. The program has two parts: hospital insurance (Part A) and medical insurance (Part B). Part B is also known as supplementary medical insurance (SMI). [1]

Merger. The resulting condition after one business, corporation, or hospital secures the capital stock of another business. The merged corporation stock is usually then dissolved. [25]

Morbidity & Mortality Committee. Reviews unusual deaths and patterns in death. [20]

Morgue. That area in a hospital where patients who have died are housed. It is usually connected to an autopsy room. [11]

Multi-Hospital System. A central association that owns and/or leases or controls, by contract, two or more hospitals. Some of the benefits of such a system are: easier availability of capital markets, mutual purchasing for greater economies of scale, and mutual use of technical and management personnel. There are two types of multi-hospital systems not-for-profit (which includes church-affiliated) or investor-owned, for profit. (Synonym: Multis) [3]

Narcotics & Barbiturates. Medications that are under the control of the Drug Enforcement Administration (DEA). (Synonym: Controlled Substances) [12]

National Resident Matching Program. Official plan and process for placement of medical school graduates into their first year of graduate medical education. The program matches the preferences of medical students for certain internships and residencies with available hospital positions. The matching process is carried out under complete confidentiality. It is frequently called "the match." [9]

Not-for-Profit Hospital. An institution defined as a non-proprietary hospital. Not-for-profit hospitals include state and local government-owned facilities. (Synonym: Voluntary Hospital) [2]

Nuclear Medicine. The field of medicine concerned with the diagnostic, therapeutic, and investigative use of radioactive compounds. Sometimes it is considered a sub-specialty of radiology. [11]

Nurse. A registered nurse (RN) or licensed practical nurse (LPN). The term usually refers to an RN, who has more education and responsibility than an LPN. [10]

Nurse Scheduling. The process in nursing management of determining when and what nursing personnel will be on duty each shift. The schedule usually applies for a specified period of time (four to six weeks) and is tailored to each individual nursing unit's needs. The needs are often determined by a patient classification, acuity, system. [10]

Nurse Staffing. The process in nursing management primarily concerned with budgeting the correct amount of nursing hours needed to adequately staff a particular nursing unit. [10]

Nurses' Station. That part of a nursing unit serving as the section focal point of administration, record keeping, and communication. Often this is where patient records for the entire nursing unit are kept. [10]

Nursing. "The diagnosis and treatment of human responses to actual or potential health problems" (American Nurses Association). It is the act of providing nursing care to patients, their families, and, in the broader sense, communities. Some nursing care activities may be performed by licensed practical nurses and nurses' aides. The hospital nursing function is organized under a Nursing Service Department, headed by a Director of Nursing, or Vice President of Nursing. [10]

Nursing, Primary Care. A system in which a professional nurse in collaboration with other members of a nursing team assumes responsibility and accountability for total care of a group of patients. [10]

Nursing Service Department. That department responsible for providing nursing care to meet patients' physical and psychological needs and to collaborate with patients' physicians in developing and implementing patient treatment plans.[10]

Nursing Staffing Standard. A standard providing a frame of reference for proper nurse staffing on a patient unit. These staffing standards are usually expressed in terms of nursing hours per patient day. (Synonym: Nursing Norm) [10]

Nursing Supervisor. A registered nurse who supervises or directs the activities of two or more nursing units. A nursing supervisor usually manages and directs the nursing services activities during the evenings, nights, and weekends. (Synonym: Patient Care Coordinator) [10]

Nursing, Team. A team, composed of registered or graduate nurses, practical nurses, aides, and orderlies, providing bedside nursing care to a group of patients under the supervision of a team leader who is a registered nurse. [10]

Nursing Unit. That geographical section, division, or area of a hospital at which the nursing organization functions. In hospitals, these geographic divisions are often located on nursing or patient floors and may be arranged along medical/surgical specialty lines. The nursing personnel in charge of these units are called head nurses or nurse managers. They report to a nursing supervisor or assistant director of nursing, or in some cases, directly to the director of nursing. While there is a variety of sizes and shapes of nursing units, most have somewhere between 20 and 40 inpatient beds. [10]

Occupancy Rate. A measure of inpatient hospital use. The ratio of inpatient beds occupied to inpatient beds available for occupancy. [2]

Occupational Therapist (OT). A registered professional trained to work with individuals who have experienced physical injuries or illnesses, psychological or developmental problems, or problems associated with the aging process. An OT requires a bachelor's degree in occupational therapy. [12]

Operating Budget. A financial plan detailing estimated income and expenses for a given time period, usually a fiscal year. Proposed income is classified by revenue sources; proposed expenses are accounted for by natural classification, such as salaries, benefits, and supplies. [17]

Osteopath (D.O.). A physician similar to an M.D. but who has graduated from a school of Osteopathic Medicine. [9]

Outpatient. A patient receiving ambulatory care at a hospital or other health facility without being admitted as an inpatient. [2, 6]

Outpatient Department. An organized unit of a hospital where outpatient services are delivered. This would include general and specialty hospital clinics. [2, 6]

Outreach. The process by which a hospital interacts with its surrounding communities. This may involve meeting community or patient needs, locating new services within the community, or offering educational health and wellness programs in addition to medical care programs. Hospitals may assign personnel to work in outreach activities. [25]

Parent Company. A separate corporate and legal entity/organization used by health care organizations for a variety of reasons, among them to react to opportunities in the marketplace. Hospitals form holding companies by a process of corporate reorganization. (Synonym: Holding Company, Foundation) [3]

Part A of Medicare. Refers to the Title XVIII of Health Insurance for the Aged of the Society Security Act, Public Law 89-97, which became effective July 1, 1966, and applies to services rendered by a provider (e.g., hospital) to an eligible beneficiary. This part is commonly referred to as hospital insurance. [16]

Part B of Medicare. Refers to Title XVIII of Health Insurance for the Aged of the Social Security Act, Public Law 89-97, which became effective July 1, 1966, and applies to services rendered by a physician to an eligible beneficiary. This part is commonly referred to as supplementary medical insurance. [16]

Pathological Services. Services performed in both clinical and anatomical pathology including microbiological, serological, chemical, hematological, biophysical, cytological, immunohematological, and pathological examinations performed on materials derived from the human body. These examinations provide information for the diagnosis, prevention, or treatment of a disease or assessment of a medical condition. (Synonym: Pathology Department, Clinical Laboratories) [11]

Patient Accounts and Billing Department. The department (traditionally referred to as the business office) responsible for managing patient accounts, hospital receivables, and patient bills. [18]

Patient Day. A unit of measure denoting room and board facilities and services provided during one 24-hour period to an inpatient. The number of such days in a month are called Patient Days Per Month. [17]

Patient Representative. An individual who works with patients, their families, hospital departments and staff, medical staff, and administration in investigating patient complaints and problems with a patient's hospital care. (Synonym: Ombudsman) [13]

Patient's Bill of Rights. An outline of the treatment and care a patient has the right to expect during hospitalization. The American Hospital Association has furnished a 12-point bill of rights as a guideline to hospitals which the hospitals can modify to accommodate local laws or customs. [8]

Pediatric Unit. A hospital clinical care unit with facilities, equipment, and personnel for the care of infants, children, and adolescents, excluding obstetrical and newborn care. [6]

Peer Review Organization (PRO). A federally funded organization established by the Social Security Act of 1983 that performs utilization and quality review in order to monitor hospitals and physicians. The organization also monitors all health care services provided to Medicare beneficiaries. Peer Review Organizations replaced the Professional Standards Review Organizations (PSROs) established in 1972. [20]

Personal Computer (PC). The computer system which is smaller than a minicomputer and differs in price, size, storage capacity, speed of execution, and computing power. [18]

Pharmacy. The art, science, and practice of preparing, preserving, compounding and dispensing drugs, as well as giving appropriate instructions for and monitoring their use. Also a location (place) where pharmaceuticals are prepared and dispensed. (Synonym: Apothecary) [12]

Pharmacy and Therapeutic Committee. A committee of hospital medical staff personnel concerned with the development and monitoring of pharmacy and therapeutic policies and practices, particularly drug utilization within a hospital. The committee generally includes the hospital pharmacists. [12]

Physical Therapist (PT). A registered professional who plans and administers physical therapy treatment programs for medically referred patients to restore function, release pain, and prevent disability following disease, injury, or loss of body parts. PTs use the treatment modalities of electricity, heat, cold, ultrasound, massage, and exercise. The educational preparation is a bachelor's or master's degree. [12]

Physiatrist. That specialty physician trained in physical medicine and rehabilitation who is responsible for the physical medicine and/or physical therapy departments. [12]

Physician. Any individual with a medical doctorate degree, M.D. or D.O. [9]

Physician's Assistant (PA). An individual who extends the service of a supervising physician by taking medical histories, performing physical examinations, and in circumscribed areas, diagnosing and treating patients. [9]

Preadmission Certification. Review and approval of the necessity and appropriateness for proposed inpatient service. The term also refers to actual admission to an institution prior to the proposed admission time. [8]

Preadmission Testing (PAT). Diagnostic tests performed in hospital outpatient areas prior to a patient's admission to the hospital. This system is used to verify the need for a hospital admission and/or reduce the inpatient's length of stay. [8]

Preferred Provider Arrangement (PPA). A direct contractual arrangement among hospitals, physicians, insurers, employers, or third-party administrators in which providers join together to offer health care for a distinct group of people. These contracts normally have three distinguishing features in common: discounts from standard charges, monetary goals for single subscribers (insurers) to utilize contracting providers, and broad utilization review programs. (Synonym: Preferred Provider Organization) [16]

Private Practice. A medical practice wherein both the practitioner and the practice are independent of any external policy control. [25]

Privileges, Clinical. A permission granted to physicians and selected other practitioners enabling them to render specific diagnostic, therapeutic, medical, dental, podiatric, or surgical services within the hospital. [9]

Privileged Communication. Statements made to a physician, attorney, spouse, or anyone else in a position of trust. Such communication is protected by law and cannot be revealed without the permission of the parties involved. [19]

Professional Standards Review Organization (PSRO). An organization created by the Social Security Amendments of 1972 which the then Department of Health, Education and Welfare charged with the responsibility of operating professional review systems to determine whether hospital services were medically necessary, provided properly, carried out on a timely basis, and met with professional standards. It was conceived as a nationwide network of locally based physicians' groups. It was disbanded in 1983 due to excessive operating costs and little documented impact on patient care. [20]

Prospective Payment System (PPS). A method of payment to hospitals in which rates for services are established in advance based on a DRG system or some other methodology. [1, 16]

Psychiatric Hospital. A specialty institution primarily concerned with providing inpatient and outpatient care and treatment for the mentally ill. [2]

Public Relations (PR). Developing goodwill with specific publics. In the hospital, the public can include patients, physicians, employees, business and industry, and the community. [20]

Purchasing Department. That department of a hospital responsible for the evaluation and procurement of the institution's supplies and specified equipment. (Synonym: Procurement Department) [15]

Quality Care. The degree to which patient care services increase the probability of desired patient outcomes. [20]

Quality Assurance (QA). Actions taken to assure quality medical and nursing care. Third-party payers and agencies frequently initiate, encourage, or mandate the establishment of such programs. [20]

Quality Assurance Program (QAP). An institutional program which generally involves a continuous process and regular review of the quality of patient care provided by the institution. [20]

Radiation Therapy. A form of medical treatment using ionizing radiation to destroy cancer and other tumors or neoplasm with minimal damage to surrounding healthy tissue. (Synonym: Radiotherapy) [11]

Radiology. The branch of medicine dealing with the use of x-rays and other forms of radiant energy in the diagnosis and treatment of disease. (Synonym: X-ray, Medical Imaging) [11]

Radiology Department. That unit in a hospital specifically designed, equipped, and staffed to use x-rays and other radioactive elements for the diagnosis and treatment of patients. This department is under the direct supervision of a radiologist (physician). This department could also include radiation therapy and/or nuclear medicine sections. (Synonym: X-ray Department, Medical Imaging Department) [11]

Reasonable Cost. Costs approved by third-party payers for reimbursement to a hospital, which are then included as a hospital's allowable costs determined by cost report. (Synonym: Cost Reimbursement, Total Cost) [16]

Rehabilitative Medicine. Medical specialty concerned with the diagnosis and treatment of certain musculoskeletal defects and neuromuscular diseases including physical therapy, occupational therapy, speech therapy, and closely related specialties. [12]

Residency. Any training following graduation from an approved medical college which leads to certification in a specialty field of medicine. This training must be approved by the American Medical Association or the American Osteopathic Association. [9]

Resident. A physician who has completed an internship or last year of medical school and is taking further supervised full-time hospital training in a specialty area of medicine. (Synonym: House Staff, Post Graduate Year (PGY)) [9]

Respiratory Care Department. An organizational unit of a hospital designed to provide ventilatory support and associated services to patients. (Synonym: Respiratory Therapy Department, Inhalation Therapy Department) [12]

Risk Management. The science of identifying, studying and controlling risks to patients, employees, and the hospital. An early warning system for identifying potential causes of liability. [21]

Risk Management Committee. One of a hospital's quality assurance committees. The committee develops policies and procedures to enhance a safe environment, conducts surveillance programs to monitor all adverse occurrences, and reviews incidence reports. [21]

Room and Board. A hospital revenue category that includes revenue from room, board, and general nursing services. (Synonym: Routine Services or Daily Patient Services; Daily Room and Board) [17]

School of Nursing. A broad term used today as a catch-all phrase for various forms of education offered to individuals pursuing a nursing career. [10]

Security Department. That unit or department of a hospital responsible for protecting patients, their families, and hospital staff as well as safeguarding the facility, equipment, and supplies. [14]

Self Pay. Individuals, institutions or corporations assuming the entire responsibility for payment of hospital and medical bills which otherwise might be covered by an insurance policy. (Synonym: Self-Insured) [16]

Semi-Private Accommodations. Accommodations provided in a room of two or more beds (usually three or four) with a charge that would generally be less than private or single bed accommodations. [10]

Shared Purchasing. A co-op arrangement between hospitals to reduce the cost of purchases. (Synonym: Group Purchasing) [16]

Skilled Nursing Facilities (SNF). Facilities providing long-term care to individuals requiring nursing care but not hospitalization. They include extended care facilities reimbursable by Medicare as well as nursing homes reimbursable by Medicaid. [2, 10]

Social Security Administration (SSA). Founded in 1946. This is the bureau of the Federal Government that is responsible for the administration of Medicare, whose financing is under the direction of the Health Care Financing Administration (HCFA). The SSA is also responsible for administering a number of other programs including the Old Age Survivors and Disability Insurance Program.

Social Service Department. That hospital unit responsible for working with patients, their families, and the institution's professional staff to assist patients with personal, socio-economic, and environmental problems related to their medical conditions. [13]

Special Diets. Foods or menus specially planned and prepared for individuals who need nutritional therapy to improve their overall health or to control disease. Such diets are usually prescribed for a patient by a physician. Type of special diets can include: modifications in consistency (liquid, soft), or content (sodium or fat restricted, high/low calorie/protein, and diabetic). [13]

Speech Therapist. A professional, registered therapist who evaluates, diagnoses, and counsels individuals with communication disorders. [13]

Student Nurses. Individuals preparing for careers as licensed practical nurses (LPNs) or registered nurses (RNs). In addition to classroom studies, nursing students must complete many hours of "hands-on" clinical training in a variety of settings. They are closely supervised by both experienced nurses and instructors as they perform routine patient care activities. Nursing schools usually contract with hospitals, nursing homes, and other health care institutions to provide clinical training sites for their students. [10]

Tax Equity and Fiscal Responsibility Act of 1982 (TEFRA). Public law 97-248, which covers many far-reaching Medicare amendments as applied to hospital reimbursement policies. This law was a first step in placing hospitals on a prospective pricing system (PPS) rather than the previous cost reimbursed, retrospective cost system. [16]

Tax Exempt Revenue Bonds. A source of debt financing for hospitals with two major features: the interest received by bond holders is not subject to federal income tax, and the organization receiving the financing secures the bonds with its gross revenues. [17]

Teaching Hospital. A hospital providing undergraduate or graduate medical education, usually with one or more medical or dental internships and/or residency programs in affiliation with a medical school. [9]

Tertiary Medicare Care. Highly sophisticated diagnostic and therapeutic services given to patients with complex and serious medical conditions. This type of care is usually rendered at teaching hospitals or at university-affiliated hospitals. [25]

Third-Party Payer. Any agency or organization which pays or insures a specific package of health or medical expenses on behalf of the beneficiaries or recipients. (Blue Cross/Blue Shield plans, Medicare, Medicaid, and Health Maintenance Organizations (HMOs) are examples). [16]

Unit Clerk. The individual who performs routine clerical or reception work on a nursing unit including receiving patients and visitors, scheduling appointments, working with records, and assisting in communications. [10]

Urgent Admission. That patient requiring admission to the hospital for a clinical condition that would require admission for diagnosis and treatment within 48 hours; otherwise the patient's life or well being could be threatened. The other two categories for admission are emergency or elective. [8]

Urgent Care Center. A freestanding facility providing minor emergency (not life-threatening) care, or basic health services on a non-scheduled basis. (Synonyms: Urgicenter; "Doc in the Box," Freestanding Emergency Room, Walk-In Clinic) [6]

Utilization. A quantitative measure of the actual use of equipment, facilities, programs, services, and personnel. This measure can be a simple rate, such as the number of admissions per day for a particular unit, or the complex evaluation of an institution's efficiency in allocating its resources, known as utilization review (UR). [20]

Utilization Review (UR). The process of examining the appropriate need of a patient's hospital admission, services provided, the patient's length of stay (LOS), and the hospital's discharge practices. This type of review is required by the JCAHO, Medicare, Medicaid, and many other third-party payers and regulatory agencies. [20]

Utilization Review Committee. A committee of the medical staff or of the hospital composed of physicians, nurses, administrative representatives, and allied health personnel. The committee's function is to review inpatients' medical records and those patients who have been discharged in order to determine the medical necessity for their treatment and hospital stay. This committee may also be involved in reviewing the discharge plans for hospitalized patients. This committee is one element in a hospital's quality assurance program. [20]

Vice President/Assistant Administrator. An individual, holding an upper level management position in a hospital, responsible for certain discrete segments, units or functions within the hospital. This person reports directly to the hospital administrator, President/CEO or the associate administrator. [5]

Volunteer. An individual who works without financial compensation performing a variety of hospital tasks within various departments. Members of the hospital auxiliary are volunteers. [15]

Volunteers, Director of. That individual, frequently a department head, who organizes and directs the training and utilization of volunteers within a hospital. This includes recruiting, assigning, and coordinating volunteers in their work assignments, and maintaining records of volunteer hours worked and the types of services performed. [15]

Index

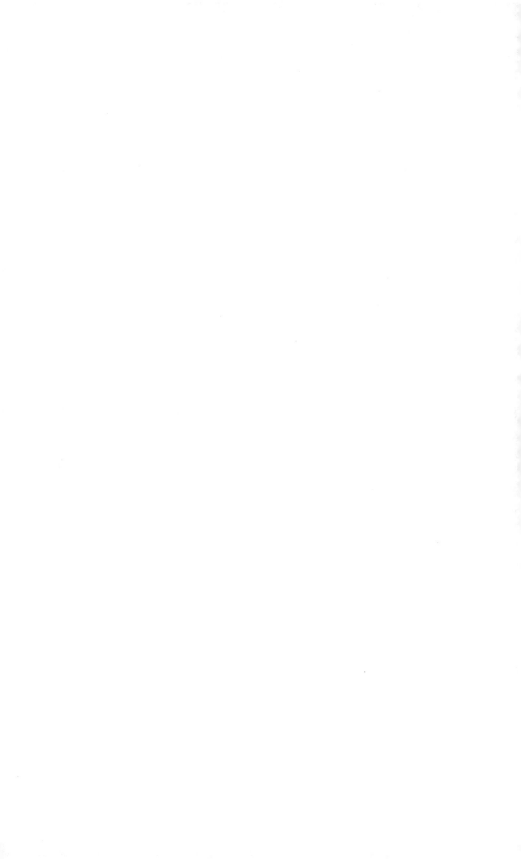